AF323610

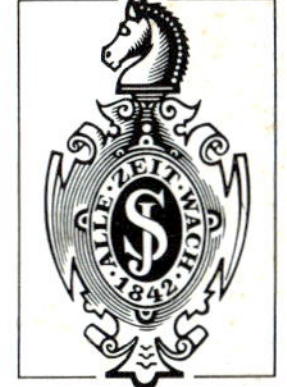

BG Chemie

Toxicological Evaluations

2 Potential Health Hazards of Existing Chemicals

Springer-Verlag

Berlin Heidelberg New York
London Paris Tokyo
Hong Kong Barcelona
Budapest

Berufsgenossenschaft
der chemischen Industrie
Gaisbergstraße 11

W-6900 Heidelberg 1, FRG

ISBN 3-540-53435-0 Springer Verlag Berlin Heidelberg New York
ISBN 0-387-53435-0 Springer Verlag New York Berlin Heidelberg

Library of Congress Cataloging-in-Publication Data. (Revised for volume 2).
Toxicological evaluations. Includes biblographical references and index. 1.
Toxicity testing. I. Berufsgenossenschaft der Chemischen Industrie. [DNLM:
1. Hazardous Substances – toxicity. WA 465 T7549]   RA1199.T678 1990
615.9'07   90-10020
ISBN 3-540-52577-7 ISBN 0-387-52577-7 (v. 1: alk. paper)
ISBN 3-540-53435-0 ISBN 0-387-53435-0 (v. 2: alk. paper)

Typesetting, printing and bookbinding: Brühlsche Universitätsdruckerei,
Giessen
51/3130-543210 – Printed on acid-free paper

Preface

As part of its programme for the prevention of health hazards caused by industrial work substances, the Berufsgenossenschaft der chemischen Industrie (BG Chemie) began in 1977 to investigate the toxicity of those substances which are widely used, have many different applications and are suspected of being dangerous to health, in particular of having long-term effects on health. It is hoped by means of this testing to close gaps in our knowledge and to increase the scientific validity of the required risk assessments. The results of the toxicological investigations carried out by BG Chemie, and the resulting substance assessments have been published in West Germany since 1987 in the form of "Toxicological Evaluations".

In order to make this useful information internationally available, the second volume (containing individual evaluations of 15 substances) is now being published in English. The first volume containing individual evaluations of 19 substances was published in October 1990. Because of the short time between publishing volumes 1 and 2, printing of the "Introduction" (consisting of a general overview of the programme, lists with names of people involved as well as substances under investigation was abandoned in volume 2. If there more detailed information is required, see volume 1 or contact BG Chemie at first hand. The publication of further individual evaluations and, if necessary, reassessments of previously published evaluations is planned.

BG Chemie hopes that, for many people working in the chemical industry, this information will be of practical help in assessing hazards to health at the workplace.

Contents

Name of substance	CAS-No.	Page
Vinyl fluoride	75-02-5	1
Methylbutadiene-1,3 (Isoprene)	78-79-5	13
Acrylic acid	79-10-7	39
o-Phthalodinitrile	91-15-6	75
m-Nitroaniline	99-09-2	87
5-Nitro-2-aminotoluene	99-52-5	101
p-Nitrosophenol	104-91-6	107
Propargyl alcohol	107-19-7	121
Diethanolamine	111-42-2	135
2-Methylpropene	115-11-7	153
2-Ethylhexanal	123-05-7	161
Maleic acid dimethyl ester	624-48-6	169
Trimethylquinone	935-92-2	177
2,4-Dinitromethylaniline	2044-88-4	185
1,5-Naphthylene diamine	2243-62-1	191
Compound chemical index vol. 1 and 2		207

Vinyl fluoride

1. Summary and assessment

After inhalation, vinyl fluoride is rapidly absorbed and distributed around the body, and is relatively slowly metabolised, probably via an epoxide intermediate. There is a transient increase in the excretion of free fluoride in the urine of rats after vinyl fluoride inhalation.

Vinyl fluoride is virtually non-toxic in acute and subchronic inhalation studies.

The available results of tests on the genotoxicity of vinyl fluoride in the Salmonella/microsome test, in *E. coli,* in CHO-cells and in the micronucleus test indicate mutagenic activity.

The similarity in biotransformation between vinyl fluoride and vinyl chloride and -bromide, together with the finding of preneoplastic foci in the livers of new-born rats after inhalation of vinyl fluoride for up to 14 weeks, suggests that the substance has carcinogenic potential. After 10-week inhalation exposure to 2000 ppm vinyl chloride, the incidence of preneoplastic foci in the liver is roughly 20 times higher than that after exposure to the same concentration of vinyl fluoride. This may be related to the rate of metabolism of vinyl fluoride, which is about 16-fold less.

The U.S. Environmental Protection Agency (EPA) has requested further mutagenicity tests and a long-term inhalation study in rats and mice to clarify the possible cancer risk.

In man, no adverse effects on health have been demonstrated at workroom air concentrations of 2 ppm (TWA) with peak levels of up to 21 ppm. Less precise documentary evidence indicates that vinyl fluoride produces nausea, dizziness and unconsciousness in man.

2. Name of substance

2.1	Usual name	Vinyl fluoride
2.2	IUPAC-name	Fluoroethylene
2.3	CAS-No.	75-02-5

3.   Synonyms common and trade names

Vinyl fluoride
Fluoroethene
Monofluoroethylene
VF

4.   Structural and molecular formulae

4.1 Structural formula $H_2C{=}CHF$

4.2 Molecular formula C_2H_3F

5.   Physical and chemical properties

5.1 Molecular mass, g/mol   46.05

5.2 Melting point, °C   −160

5.3 Boiling point, °C   −72

5.4 Vapour pressure, hPa   25,000 (at 21 °C)

5.5 Density, g/cm³   0.636 (at 20 °C under pressure)

5.6 Solubility in water   insoluble

5.7 Solubility in organic solvents   soluble in alcohol dimethylformamide, ether

5.8 Solubility in fat   no information available

5.9 pH-value   −

5.10 Conversion factor   1 ppm $\hat{=}$ 1.91 mg/m³
1 mg/m³ $\hat{=}$ 0.52 ppm
(at 25 °C and 1013 hPa)
(Du Pont, 1969; Hommel, 1988; Kühn-Birett, 1976)

6.   Uses

Manufacture of polyvinylfluoride and related copolymers (von Halasz and Millauer, 1976).

7.   Experimental results

7.1   Toxicokinetics and metabolism

On exposure of male Wistar rats to vinyl fluoride at a concentration of 100 ppm (191 mg/m^3), a concentration equilibrium forms between the atmosphere and the organism within 30 minutes. The following values have been given as equilibrium constants K_{eq} for the distribution of the test substances vinyl fluoride (VF), vinyl chloride (VC) and vinyl bromide (VBr) between the inhalation chamber and the animal body:

VF K_{eq} =   0.91
VC K_{eq} =   5.3
VBr K_{eq} = 11.3.

It is evident from these values that there is a close relationship between the K_{eq}-value and the volatility and boiling point of the vinyl halogens. Thus, due to its low boiling point, vinyl fluoride accumulates to only a small extent in the tissues. A maximum metabolic rate of 7 µmol/h×kg body weight was reached in rats at an atmospheric concentration of about 75 ppm (143.3 mg/m^3) vinyl fluoride (saturation point, SP). At this concentration, the metabolism follows first order kinetics.

Table 1. Metabolism

Substance	SP ppm in air	Clearance 1st order 1/h × kg	Zero order V_{max} µmol/h × kg
VF	75[a]	2.5	7
VC	250	11.0	110
VBr	55	18	40

[a] Estimated

According to these data, vinyl fluoride is very slowly metabolised under saturation conditions (Filser and Bolt, 1979, 1981).

In a later pharmacokinetic investigation, male Wistar rats whose metabolic capacity was saturated (2000 ppm = 3822 mg/m^3, V_{max}-conditions) were exposed to concentrations of vinyl fluoride in a closed system. An increase in acetone exhalation during the 50-hour observation period occurred with vinyl fluoride and likewise with vinyl chloride. It could not be elucidated whether the acetonaemia in rats inhaling vinyl fluoride and other halogenated ethylene compounds was metabolically caused, or whether other mechanisms were involved (Filser et al., 1982).

Male Sprague-Dawley rats (200–225 g) inhaled 3000 ppm (5733 mg/m^3) vinyl fluoride for 30 minutes and were then held for 14 days in metabolic chambers (2 groups, five animals each). Fluoride concentrations in 24-hour urine samples were measured over a period of 14 days. The urinary levels of glucose, protein and blood were determined, as was the pH value (using reagent strips). Sodium and potassium contents were measured by flame photometry and creatinine content by Technikon-autoanalyser. A further group of five rats was examined microscopically and macroscopically at fixed time intervals. Fluoride excretion in the urine (at 3.77±0.23 µmol) was significantly increased (p <0.01) compared to the controls (1.71±0.14 µmol) six days after exposure. In addition, the volume of urine was significantly increased (p <0.05) on the 2nd day (9.3±0.4 ml), the 5th day (10.7±0.6 ml), the 7th day (11.1±1.2 ml), the 12th day (13.0±0.7 ml) and the 14th day (12.9±1.6 ml; controls: 7.6±0.8 ml, 9.2±0.5 ml, 8.1±0.7 ml, 10.8±0.6 ml and 11.1±4.4 ml respectively). The daily potassium excretion was similarly significantly increased (p <0.01) on the 2nd day at 4.89±0.14 mEq (controls 4.32±0.20 mEq) and on the 6th day at 4,98±0.06 mEq (controls 4.29±0.34 mEq). The other parameters remained unaffected. Histologically, there were pathological changes in the kidney (hyperaemia of the kidney medulla, pale whitish bands in the kidney cortex) which were most severe 3–4 days after exposure and were almost reversed after 2 weeks (Dilley et al., 1974).

Comparative investigations have shown that in rats vinyl fluoride is metabolised about 16 times slower than vinyl chloride. After 10 weeks of exposure at 2000 ppm (3822 mg/m^3, 8 hours/day, 5 days/week) rates of metabolism were 110 µmol/hour/kg body weight for vinyl chloride and 7 µmol/hour/kg body weight for vinyl fluoride (Bolt et al., 1982).

7.2   Acute and subacute toxicity

Vinyl fluoride is only of low acute inhalation toxicity to white rats (no details of strain and sex) even at high concentrations. No deaths occurred after a 30-minute exposure period at concentrations of 10–80% (no information on the number of animals). Enriched oxygen supplies were ensured in these studies. Paralysis of the hind limbs was observed in animals exposed to 30% vinyl fluoride; at 60% vinyl fluoride the stopping reflex was no longer demonstrable; at 70%, the postural reflex disappeared; at 80%, the corneal reflex was still present, but dyspnoea occurred. The experimental animals recovered within a short time of transfer to pure air. Histopathological investigation did not reveal any damage to the lungs. A few animals (number not given) were exposed to 80% vinyl fluoride for up to 12.5 hours. The corneal reflex was retained for the entire period. These rats also recovered immediately after being brought into a normal atmosphere. Their lungs showed no signs of irritation (Lester and Greenberg, 1950).

Mice (NMRI-SPF (Han/Bö), 7–8 weeks old, 20 of each sex) survived inhalation exposure to a mixture of 80% vinyl fluoride and 20% oxygen for 8 hours. Observed symptoms of toxicity included scratching, convulsions, disturbance of balance and salivation. The symptoms disappeared completely within 24 hours (Otto, 1982).

Groups of between three and seven male Holtzmann rats were treated with polychlorinated biphenyls (PCB, Aroclor 1254, 300 μmol/kg, by stomach tube) on 3 consecutive days. They were then exposed to vinyl fluoride by inhalation for 4 hours at a concentration of 10,000 ppm (19,100 mg/m^3). Liver damage and increased levels of serum alanine-α-ketoglutarate transaminase and sorbitol dehydrogenase were seen (Conolly et al., 1978; Conolly and Jaeger, 1977). When rats received a single dose of trichloropropane epoxide (epoxide-hydrase inhibitor) by stomach tube (1 ml/kg as a 10% solution) immediately before the inhalation study, two of the six normally-fed animals, and one of the six fasted rats died (Conolly and Jaeger, 1977).

Rats exposed to various vinyl fluoride concentrations (5000, 10,000, 35,000, 102,000 ppm $\hat{=}$ 9560, 19,100, 66,890, 194,920 mg/m^3) after PCB pre-treatment showed signs of liver damage (increased serum alanine-α-ketoglutarate transaminase, increased liver weight) when compared with PCB-treated controls (not exposed to vinyl fluoride). These effects were dose-dependent up to 10,000 ppm (19,100 mg/m^3), but a plateau was reached at higher concentrations. At concentrations of 102,000 ppm (194,920 mg/m^3) four out of seven rats died, the deaths occurring 4–24 hours after the beginning of the experiment. Histopathological examination of the liver revealed swelling of the hepatocytes and centro-lobular necroses. Similar results were obtained with vinyl chloride (investigated at the same time for comparative purposes) at concentrations of 10,000, 24,000 and 50,000 ppm (Conolly et al., 1978).

7.3   Skin and mucous membrane effects

No information available.

7.4   Sensitization

No information available.

7.5   Subchronic and chronic toxicity

Rats exposed by inhalation for 7 hours/day, 5 days per week for 6 weeks to 100,000 ppm (191,000 mg/m^3) vinyl fluoride (no details of strain or number of animals), showed no symptoms of toxicity after clinical observation, monitoring of body-weight gain, macro- and micropathological examination and measurement of organ weight (Du Pont, 1969).

7.6   Genotoxicity

7.6.1 In vitro

In the Salmonella/microsome test, strains TA 98, TA 100, TA 1535, TA 1537, and TA 1538 were exposed to an atmosphere of 80% vinyl fluoride and 20% oxygen in a closed system. The test was carried out with and without metabolic activation (S9 from Aroclor-induced rat liver). Vinyl fluoride has no demonstrable bacteriotoxic effect. Mutagenic activity was not detectable either with or without metabolic activation in strains TA 98, TA 1537, and TA 1538. Increased numbers of revertants were seen in the presence of a metabolic activation system in strains TA 100 and TA 1535, the increases being by factors of 1.4 and 3–4, respectively. No effect could be detected in either strain without metabolic activation (Spiegelberg, 1983).

Vinyl fluoride was tested for gene mutations in the CHO-HGPRT test, and proved to be negative without metabolic activation and positive with metabolic activation (no further details; Du Pont, 1986a).

In the chromosome aberration test with CHO-cells, the activity of vinyl fluoride without metabolic activation was questionable, while positive results were obtained with metabolic activation (no further details; Du Pont, 1986b).

Gassing a liquid culture of *Escherichia coli* B for 10 minutes with vinyl fluoride leads to a change in carbohydrate metabolism (Landry and Fuerst, 1968). It is not clear whether the apparent effect of vinyl fluoride on the citric acid cycle is due to a (biochemical) mutation or due to cytotoxicity.

7.6.2 In vivo

To investigate micronucleus formation, 43-day-old male and female Crl:CD-1 (ICR) BR mice were exposed to vinyl fluoride (purity 99.99%) by inhalation for 6 hours at concentrations of 50,100 ppm (95, 740 mg/m^3), 191,000 ppm (365,000 mg/m^3) or 388,000 ppm (741,500 mg/m^3). The polychromatic erythrocytes of the bone marrow were examined for micronuclei at 24, 48 and 72 hours after the beginning of exposure. Cyclophosphamide served as a positive control. After 24 hours the females exposed to 191,000 and 388,000 ppm showed a statistically-significant dose-dependent increase in micronuclei in the polychromatic erythrocytes. In male mice at the same two concentrations, the frequency of micronuclei was also increased, but the findings were not statistically significant. 48 and 72 hours after the beginning of exposure, the micronuclei of the exposed mice at all concentrations and in both sexes did not differ from those of the controls (Du Pont, 1987).

The US Environmental Protection Agency has asked for mutagenicity tests to be conducted with vinyl fluoride in a step-wise approach (Drosophila test, mouse-specific locus assay, dominant lethal test, heritable translocation assay; US EPA, 1987).

7.7 Carcinogenicity

There is no literature available on the carcinogenic activity of vinyl fluoride in mature experimental animals. However, pre-neoplastic hepatocellular foci have been found in young Wistar rats exposed to a vinyl fluoride concentration of 2000 ppm (3822 mg/m^3) for 8 hours/day, 5 days/week from the day of birth up to the age of 14 weeks. Unexposed controls showed no pre-neoplastic liver foci after 14 weeks, but in treated females 0.0012% of the hepatocytes were ATP-ase deficient after 4 weeks, 0.042% after 10 weeks and 0.087% after 14 weeks. The publication does not state whether male rats were also studied (Bolt et al., 1981). The authors obtained qualitatively similar results after equivalent studies with vinyl chloride and vinyl bromide (Bolt, 1980; Bolt et al., 1982; Bolt et al., 1979).

The US Environmental Protection Agency has urgently requested chronic inhalation studies in rats and mice for clarification of possible carcinogenic potential (US EPA, 1987).

7.8 Reproductive toxicity

No information available.

7.9 Effects on the immune system
No information available.

7.10 Neurotoxicity
No information available.

7.11 Other effects
No information available.

8.   Experience in humans

Studies in a plant manufacturing vinyl fluoride gave estimated workplace concentrations of 2 ppm (3.82 mg/m^3; TWA), with individual values of up to 21 ppm (40.13 mg/m^3; start of production). Vinyl fluoride values of 1–4 ppm (1.91–7.64 mg/m^3) were measured in a vinyl fluoride polymer manufacturing factory. Adverse effects to health would not be expected in these ranges (Oser, 1980).

According to information which cannot be further pursued, nausea, dizziness and unconsciousness can occur after exposure to vinyl fluoride, presumably as a result of displacement of breathed air (Kühn-Birett, 1976).

References

Bolt, H.M.
Die toxikologische Beurteilung halogenierter Äthylene
Arbeitsmedizin, Sozialmedizin, Präventivmedizin, 15, 49–53 (1980)

Bolt, H.M., Laib, R.J., Stöckle, G.
Formation of pre-neoplastic hepatocellular foci by vinyl bromide in newborn rats
Arch. Toxicol., 43, 83–84 (1979)

Bolt, H.M., Laib, R.J., Klein, K.P.
Formation of pre-neoplastic hepatocellular foci by vinyl fluoride in newborn rats
Arch. Toxicol., 47, 71–73 (1981)

Bolt, H.M., Laib, R.J., Filser, J.G.
Reactive metabolites and carcinogenicity of halogenated ethylenes
Biochem. Pharmacol., 31, 1–4 (1982)

Conolly, R.B., Jaeger, R.J., Szabo, S.
Acute hepatotoxicity of ethylene, vinyl fluoride, vinyl chloride and
vinyl bromide after Aroclor 1254 pretreatment
Exp. Molec. Pathol., 28, 25–33 (1978)

Conolly, R.B., Jaeger, R.J.
Acute hepatotoxicity of ethylene and halogenated ethylenes after
PCB pretreatment
Environ. Health Perspect., 21, 131–135 (1977)

Dilley, J.V., Carter, V.L., Jr., Harris, E.S.
Fluoride ion excretion by male rats after inhalation of one of several
fluoroethylenes or hexafluoropropene
Toxicol. Appl. Pharmacol., 27, 582–590 (1974)

Du Pont de Nemours, E.I. and Co.
Vinyl fluoride, vinylidene fluoride
Technical Report DP-6, Wilmington, Delaware (1969)

Du Pont de Nemours, E.I. and Co.
Mutagenicity evaluation of vinyl fluoride in the CHO/HGPRT assay
Wilmington, Delaware (1986a)
Cited by US EPA (1987)

Du Pont de Nemours, E.I. and Co.
Evaluation of vinyl fluoride in the in vitro assay from chromosome
aberrations in Chinese hamsters ovary (CHO) cells
Wilmington, Delaware (1986b)
Cited by US EPA (1987)

Du Pont de Nemours, E.I. and Co.
Mouse bone marrow micronucleus assay of vinyl fluoride
Unpublished report, Wilmington, Delaware (1987)

Filser, J.G., Bolt, H.M.
Pharmacokinetics of halogenated ethylenes in rats
Arch. Toxicol., 42, 123–136 (1979)

Filser, J.G., Bolt, H.M.
Inhalation pharmacokinetics based on gas uptake studies
1. Improvement of kinetic models
Arch. Toxicol., 47, 279–292 (1981)

Filser, J.G., Jung, P., Bolt, H.M.
Increased acetone exhalation induced by metabolites of halogenated C_1 and C_2 compounds
Arch. Toxicol., 49, 107–116 (1982)

Hommel, G. (ed.)
Handbuch der gefährlichen Güter
Data Sheet 398
Springer, Berlin Heidelberg New York, 3rd edition (1988)

Kühn-Birett
Merkblätter Gefährliche Arbeitsstoffe
Sheet No. V 04, supplement 3, 6/76 (1976)

Landry, M.M., Fuerst, R.
Gas ecology of bacteria
Dev. Ind. Microbiol., 9, 370–380 (1968)

Lester, D., Greenberg, L.A.
Acute and chronic toxicity of some halogenated derivates of methane and ethane
Arch. Ind. Hyg. Occ. Med., 2, 335–344 (1950)

Oser, J.L.
Extent of industrial exposure to epichlorohydrin, vinyl fluoride, vinyl bromide and ethylene dibromide
Am. Ind. Hyg. Ass. J., 41, 463–468 (1980)

Otto, F.
Mikronukleustest
Unpublished results from the Fraunhofer-Institut für Toxikologie und Aerosolforschung, Schmallenberg-Grafschaft (1982)
Commissioned by BG Chemie

Spiegelberg, T.
Kurzzeittest auf mutagene Wirksamkeit: Salmonella Mikrosomentest (nach Ames)
Unpublished results from the Fraunhofer-Institut für Toxikologie und Aerosolforschung, Schmallenberg-Grafschaft (1983)
Commissioned by BG Chemie

von Halasz, S.P., Millauer, H.
Fluorverbindungen, organische
in Ullmanns Enzyklopädie der technischen Chemie
Volume 11, p. 642
Verlag Chemie, Weinheim (1976)

US Environmental Protection Agency (US EPA)
Fluoroalkenes; Final Test Rule
Federal Register, Vol. 52, No. 109 of 8. 6. 1987, p. 21516–21532
(1987)

Methylbutadiene-1,3 (Isoprene)

1.   Summary and assessment

In animals, Methylbutadiene-1,3 (isoprene) and its metabolites are excreted mainly via the urine. The principal metabolites in vitro are 3,4-epoxy-3-methyl-2-butene and trans-3-methyl-1-butene-3,4-diol, but the metabolites formed in vivo have not yet been characterised. Isoprene is formed endogenously in rats, mice and humans. In rats exposed by inhalation, isoprene accumulates mainly in the perirenal fat and the subcutaneous adipose tissue. Smaller quantitites are detectable in the brain, spleen, kidneys and liver.

Isoprene is of low acute toxicity (LD_{50} rat oral 2125 mg/kg, LD_{50} rat dermal >1000 µl/kg, LC_{50} rat 180 mg/l air/4 hours (=64500 ppm)). Single or repeated inhalation exposure of mice to isoprene causes changes in the thymus and spleen (organ weight, mitotic index and, in the thymus, variable cell count). The lymphocyte count in the peripheral blood is increased. These findings indicate that isoprene has an effect on the immune system. Other effects that have also been observed include aplastic anaemia, testicular atrophy, degeneration of the olfactory epithelium and hyperplasia of the epithelium lining the forestomach. In further tests on rats involving repeated inhalation exposure (over 6 months), there was a decrease in hippuric acid formation in the liver. Histopathological examination revealed bronchitis and hyperplasia of the lungs, and histiocytic infiltration of the liver and heart.

In bacterial tests, there is no evidence that isoprene itself induces point-mutations. However, liver microsomes metabolise isoprene to 2-methyl-1,2,3,4-diepoxybutane, which is mutagenic to strains TA 98 and TA 100 in the Salmonella/microsome test. In mouse in vivo tests, isoprene induces sister chromatid exchange and micronucleus formation. Chromosome aberrations and changes in the mitotic index have not been observed.

Isoprene is not embryotoxic or teratogenic after oral administration to the rat.

In the rabbit, repeated inhalation exposure causes a reduction in non-specific immune parameters (reduced numbers of phagocytes and phagocytic index, and a shift in the albumin-globulin ratio).

Isoprene is cytotoxic to mouse bone marrow, inhibiting cell proliferation and erythropoiesis. In the Lim test no cumulative effects have been found.

In man, isoprene causes irritation of the skin, eyes and respiratory tract. Workers in the rubber industry exposed repeated, by inhalation to isoprene show a reduction in the number of phagocytes and in the phagocytic index. With increasing length of exposure, there is a corresponding increase in the incidence of upper respiratory tract irritation, together with increased incidences of influenza, angina, and diseases of the liver and gall bladder. After repeated skin contact with isoprene, workers experience itching followed by dermatitis and eczema on the backs of the hands, forearms and face. The skin becomes dry and flaky.

In the Soviet Union, a maximum limit value (TLV) of 0.04 mg/l air has been recommended.

As part of the National Toxicology Program, a 13-week and 6-month study in rats and mice is currently in progress in the USA.

2.   Name of substance

2.1 Usual name	Isoprene
2.2 IUPAC-name	2-Methyl-1,3-butadiene
2.3 CAS-No.	78-79-5

3.   Synonyms, common and trade names

Methylbutadiene-1,3
β-Methyl bivinyl
Hemiterpene

4.   Structural and molecular formulae

4.1   Structural formula

$$H_2C{=}C{-}CH{=}CH_2$$
$$|$$
$$CH_3$$

4.2   Molecular formula C_5H_8

5.   Physical and chemical properties

5.1	Molecular mass, g/mol	68.114
5.2	Melting point, °C	−145.95 (Ullmann, 1975)
5.3	Boiling point, °C	34.067 (Ullmann, 1975)
5.4	Vapour pressure, hPa	605.3 (at 20 °C) (Ullmann, 1975)
5.5	Density, g/cm^3	0.6810 (at 20 °C) (Ullmann, 1975)
5.6	Solubility in water	0.029 Mol-% ($\hat{=}$1.98 mg/100 ml) (Ullmann, 1975)
5.7	Solubility in organic solvents	Fully miscible with ethanol, diethyl ether, acetone and benzene (Ullmann, 1975)
5.8	Solubility in fat	No information available.
5.9	pH-value	−
5.10	Conversion factor	1 ppm $\hat{=}$ 2.79 mg/m^3 1 mg/m^3 $\hat{=}$ 0.36 ppm (at 25 °C and 1013 hPa) (Clayton and Clayton, 1982)
5.11	Odour threshold	3.7 ppm (Stahl, 1973)
5.12	Distribution coefficient (log Pow)	3.6 (Lyman et al., 1982)

6.   Uses

Raw material for cis-1,4-polyisoprene (IR; production of car tyres) and butyl rubber (IIR, copolymerized with isobutene; Ullmann, 1975).

7.   Experimental results

7.1   Toxicokinetics and metabolism

Isoprene is metabolised by male mouse, rat, hamster and rabbit liver microsomes in vitro in the following way:

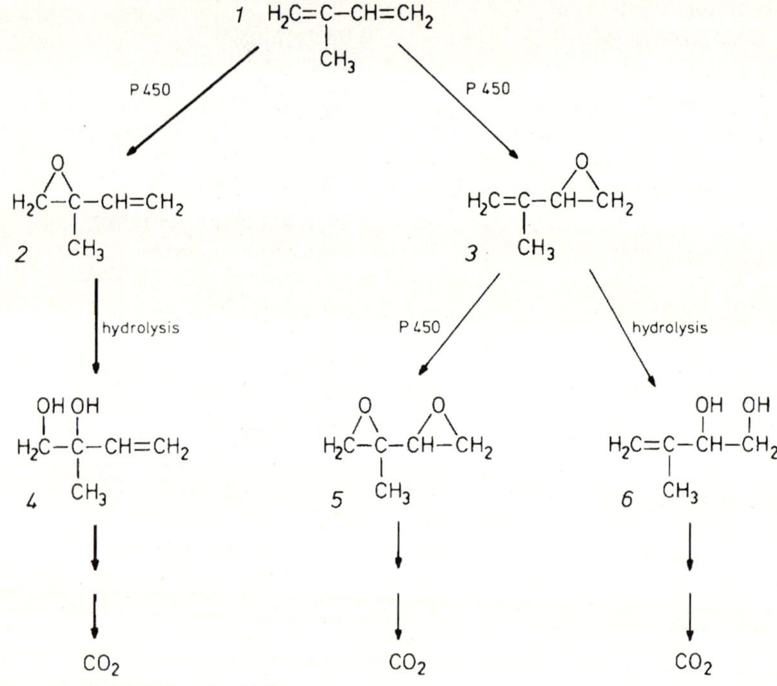

1) Isoprene
2) 3,4-Epoxy-3-methyl-1-butene ==== primary metabolism
3) 3,4-Epoxy-2-methyl-1-butene
4) trans-3-Methyl-1-butene-3,4-diol
5) 2-Methyl-1,2,3,4-diepoxybutane ——— secondary metabolism
6) trans-2-Methyl-1-butene-3,4-diol

There is no qualitative difference between non-induced and phenobarbital- or 2-methylcholanthrene-induced livers. Phenobarbital increases (p≤0.01) the metabolism of 3,4-epoxy-2-methyl-1-butene to 2-methyl-1,2,3,4-diepoxybutane, while 2-methylcholanthrene does not influence the oxidation process.

The metabolism follows Michaelis-Menten kinetics. Isoprene is metabolised in vitro mainly to 3,4-epoxy-3-methylbutene and trans-3-methyl-1-butene-3,4-diol.

The following concentration ratio between 3,4-epoxy-2-methyl-1-butene and 3,4-epoxy-3-methyl-1-butene was determined after a two-hour incubation of liver microsomes with isoprene:

Table 1. Metabolite concentrations for different species (Del Monte et al., 1985; Longo et al., 1985)

Species	Concentration ratio of 3,4-epoxy-2-methyl-1-butene to 3,4-epoxy-3-methyl-1-butene (=100 %)
Mouse	20%
Rat	25%
Hamster	17%
Rabbit	14%

In vivo. Studies on the kinetics of isoprene metabolism were carried out in F-344 rats (Dahl et al., 1987). Vacuum line cryogenic distillation was used for quantitative determination of the compounds. This method enables compounds to be identified by their freezing point, but does not permit unequivocal characterisation of the same or similar isomers, only fractions with the same freezing point. The following freezing points were determined for *in vitro* characterisation of the metabolites:

Table 2. Metabolite freezing points

Metabolite	Freezing point °C
Isoprene	−130
3,4-Epoxy-3-methyl-1-butene	− 95
3,4-Epoxy-2-methyl-1-butene	− 95
2-Methyl-1,2,3,4-diepoxybutane	− 45
trans-3-Methyl-1-butene-3,4-diol	− 45
trans-2-Methyl-1-butene-3,4-diol	− 45
CO_2	−196

The rats were exposed in nose-only inhalation chambers. Radiolabelled isoprene was used: 4-[^{14}C]-2-methyl-1,3-butadiene. Isoprene was absorbed through the respiratory tract dosedependently. Five male rats were used per group:

Table 3. Retention of inhaled isoprene

Concentration of isoprene in the air	Duration of exposure	Total isoprene inhaled during exposure	Total ^{14}C retained in rats at end of exposure	^{14}C retention[a]
(ppm)	(hours)	(μmol)	(μmol)	(%)
8 ± 0.2	6	18	3.5	19 ± 3
266 ± 10	6	736	67.1	9.1 ± 0.8
1480 ± 20	6	3650	211	5.8 ± 0.9
8200 ± 320	5.5	14200	641	4.5 ± 0.7

[a] Isoprene equivalents

After a 6-hour exposure to 1480 ppm isoprene in the air, the fractions were determined (summarised in Table 12, see appendix). The radioactivity accumulated predominantly in the liver, fat and blood, but was also found in the nasal cavity and in the lungs. Isoprene was almost completely metabolised, the main metabolites being conjugates, tetrols, diols and diepoxy-compounds. No residual isoprene was found in the tissues analysed at the end of the 18-hour observation period. There were no indications of storage or binding of isoprene metabolites. Saturation of isoprene metabolism apparently occurs between 266 and 1480 ppm on exposure for 6 hours. While no isoprene could be detected in the blood at 8 and 266 ppm, it was detectable at higher exposure concentrations (1480 and 8200 ppm), the level being dependent on the exposure concentration. A plateau concentration in the blood is also seen for the conjugate, tetrol and monoepoxides (see Table 13 in appendix). With shorter exposure periods (20 or 120 minutes) no saturation of metabolic capacity is observed (not described). The elimination of radioactivity in the urine proceeds independently of the exposure concentration.

After exposure for 6 or 5.5 hours, the radioactivity is excreted as follows (0–66 hours, n=4):

Table 4. Excretion of radioactivity

Concentration	Duration of exposure	Urine	Faeces	CO_2[a]	Carcass
(ppm)	(hours)	(% of total radioactivity absorbed)			
8	6	76.7	2.4	2.8	18.2
266	6	78.3	3.3	3.3	15.0
1480	6	81.3	1.7	1.9	16.6
8200	5.5	73.3	13.4	5.3	8.0

[a] Determined exclusively as radioactively-labelled CO_2

The half-life for elimination of radioactivity in the urine was 10.2±1.0 hours (range 8.8–11.1 hours; Dahl et al., 1987).

The saturation of isoprene metabolism was confirmed in a second study. The metabolism of isoprene in the mouse (B6C3F1) and the rat (Wistar) proceeds in proportion to the atmospheric concentration up to a level of around 300 ppm in the air. In the rat, up to a concentration of 250 ppm, 15% of the absorbed isoprene is eliminated unchanged in the exhaled air, while in the mouse, up to a concentration of 300 ppm, 25% is eliminated unchanged. At higher exposure concentrations, the proportion of isoprene eliminated in the exhaled air increases dose-dependently. The study was carried out in a closed system (desiccator). Groups of two male rats or five male mice were exposed to isoprene for $7^{1}/_2$ to 10 hours. At the beginning of the study, the concentrations were 5 to 4000 ppm. The rate of metabolism of isoprene was dependent on the exposure level. In rats, the V_{max} (maximum velocity) for the metabolism of isoprene was 130 µmol/hour/kg body weight at a concentration of about 1500 ppm, whilst in the mouse it was about 400 µmol/hour/kg body weight at around 2000 ppm (Peter et al., 1987).

This species difference had previously been observed *in vitro*. The V_{max} (nmol trans-3-Methyl-1-butene-3,4-diol/mg protein/minute) was 0.24 in rat liver microsomes and 1.79 in mouse liver microsomes (Longo et al., 1985).

At high concentrations, isoprene accumulation in the body was determined from distribution coefficients (thermodynamic partition coefficient) for isoprene and from inhalation and exhalation volumes. The calculated distribution coefficients (body/air) were 7.8 ± 3 for the rat and 7.0 ± 2 for the mouse.

Table 5. Other pharmacokinetic parameters that have also been reported (Peter et al., 1987)

	Mouse	Rat
Elimination half-life (<300 ppm)	4.4 minutes	6.8 minutes
Elimination half-life (>300 ppm)	18 minutes	44 minutes
Clearances	$12,000 \pm 3000$ ml/h	6200 ± 1000 ml/h

In a further study on the distribution of isoprene in the tissues of the rat, the following values were determined after inhalation of about 180 mg isoprene/l for 4 hours ($\hat{=}$64,500 ppm, this concentration corresponding approximately to the LC_{50} value reported in this study):

Table 6. Isoprene distribution in tissues

Organ	Isoprene Concentration (mg/l)	95% Confidence Limits	
Brain	39.5	32.1– 46.2	(n=10)
Liver	43.3	34.7– 51.9	(n=10)
Kidney	39.6	26.7– 52.5	(n=7)
Spleen	28.0	19.1– 36.9	(n=7)
Kidney capsule fat	257.7	178.4–337.1	(n=7)
Subcutaneous fat	178.4	149.0–207.8	(n=7)

According to the authors' data, this study shows a correlation between the narcotic effect and the isoprene concentration measured in the tissues (no further information, Shugaev, 1968).

In anaesthetized dogs in which breathing was artificially regulated, the retention of isoprene was independent of the frequency and volume of breathing. Five mongrels were used per study group. At an isoprene concentration of 0.40–0.60 µg/ml ($\hat{=}$143–215 ppm) retention by the respiratory organs was about 65–75%. In this study, a respiratory volume averaging 112–218 ml at 14–16 inhalations/minute and an average respiratory frequency of 6–30 inhalations/minute were recorded. The percentage retained was concentration-dependent (the respiratory frequency being 12–20 inhalations/minute):

Table 7. Isoprene retention in respiratory organs (Egle and Gochberg, 1975)

Average isoprene concentration (µg/ml)	Retention by the respiratory organs (%)
0.36 ($\hat{=}$ 129 ppm)	63.9 ± 0.82
0.51 ($\hat{=}$ 183 ppm)	72.0 ± 0.66
0.72 ($\hat{=}$ 258 ppm)	69.0± 1.02
0.96 ($\hat{=}$ 344 ppm)	39.5 ± 0.95

Based on studies carried out in the mouse, Dahl et al. (1987) calculated that the following diepoxybutane levels were the maximum blood levels that could be attained by the end of the exposure. It was assumed that the whole diol-/diepoxy-fraction consisted of 2-methyl-1,2,3,4-diepoxybutane. The calculation is based on the data in Table 13 in the appendix, assuming a blood volume of 15 ml:

Table 8. Diepoxybutane levels in mouse

Exposure concentration (ppm)	Exposure time (hours)	calculated level of 2-methyl-1,2,3,4-diepoxybutane in the blood (μ)[a]
8	6	0.37 ($\hat{=}$ 0.037 µg/ml)
266	6	7.4 ($\hat{=}$ 0.74 µg/ml)
1480	6	15.0 ($\hat{=}$ 1.50 µg/ml)
8200	5.5	17.0 ($\hat{=}$ 1.70 µg/ml)

[a] In the original publication, values were given in mM; this is obviously a misprint

It must be borne in mind that 2-methyl-1,2,3,4-diepoxybutane has not yet been unequivocally demonstrated in vivo. It may also be of significance that isoprene is formed endogenously.

Table 9. Values available for endogenous isoprene metabolism in animals (Peter et al., 1987)

	Mouse	Rat
Isoprene formation µmol/hour/kg	0.4	1.9
Metabolism µmol/hour/kg	0.31	1.6

In a further study, no isoprene could be detected in the exhaled air of the mouse, guinea-pig, rabbit, dog or chicken, but it could be detected in rats during lactation or on feeding with sour cream and cottage cheese. There is no information on the detection threshold (Gelmont et al., 1981).

7.2   Acute and subacute toxicity

Groups of 15 male and 15 female Wistar rats (weight 160 to 210 g) received single doses of 250–2500 mg isoprene/kg body weight (in oil), by stomach tube. The LD_{50} value was 2125 (2043–2210) mg/kg body weight. Observed effects included sedation and breathing difficulties, which continued up to 7 days after administration. Deaths occurred within 24 hours (Kimmerle and Solmecke, 1972).

To ascertain the LD_{50} for acute dermal application, 1000 ml isoprene/kg body weight were applied to the dorsal skin of five rats which had been shaved on the previous day. It was not removed from the skin for 7 days. An LD_{50} value of >1000 ml/kg was determined. There were no symptoms of toxicity during the observation period (Kimmerle and Solmecke, 1972).

Groups of 15 male Wistar rats (weight 160–200 g) received a single intraperitoneal injection of isoprene at dose levels of 100–1750 mg/kg body weight. An LD_{50} value of 1390 (1310–1470) mg/kg body weight was determined. The symptoms of toxicity were similar to those observed on oral adminstration (Kimmerle and Solmecke, 1972).

After single inhalation exposure of isoprene to rats and mice the following LC_{50}-values could be shown (see table 10):

Table 10. LC_{50} values for rats and mice determined on inhalation exposure to isoprene

Species	Duration of exposure	LC_{50}	95% confidence limits
Mouse	2 hours	139 mg/l ($\hat{=}$ 49,800 ppm)	135–143 mg/l ($\hat{=}$ 48,400–51,300 ppm)
Mouse	2 hours	148 mg/l ($\hat{=}$ 53,000 ppm)	144–153 mg/l ($\hat{=}$ 51,600–54,800 ppm)
Mouse[a]	2 hours	157 mg/l ($\hat{=}$ 56,300 ppm)	130–181 mg/l ($\hat{=}$ 46,600–64,900 ppm)
Mouse[a]	4 hours	214 mg/l ($\hat{=}$ 76,700 ppm)	
Rat[a]	4 hours	180 mg/l ($\hat{=}$ 64,500 ppm)	129–252 mg/l ($\hat{=}$46,200–90,300 ppm)

[a] Information on sex not available

Data on the number of animals used and the observation period are not given in the reports (Shugaev, 1969; Gostinskii, 1965; Mamedov, 1979). Dyspnoea, decreased motor activity and narcosis have been observed in rats and mice during acute inhalation exposure (Gostinskii, 1965). The surviving animals recovered within 30 minutes of the end of exposure (Shugaev, 1969). In the mouse, the threshold value for decreased motor activity is about 1.1 mg isoprene/l ($\hat{=}$ 394 ppm) for a 40 minute exposure. The EC_{50} value for a narcotic effect (loss of righting reflexes) is 109 mg/l ($\hat{=}$ 39,100 ppm) for a 2-hour exposure. At autopsy, the lungs of the mice were enlarged and congested (Gostinskii, 1965).

In a further study in the mouse, a reduced cell count and mitotic index were measured in the thymus 24 hours after exposure to concentrations of 8.40±1.09 mg/l and 21.41±1.63 mg/l for 4 hours ($\hat{=}$3011±391 and 7674±584 ppm). The absolute and relative thymus weights were also significantly reduced. Three days after exposure, the values had returned to normal. At lower isoprene concentrations (0.81 or 2.18 mg/l $\hat{=}$ 290 or 780 ppm) there were increases in the mitotic index in the thymus and in the number of lymphocytes in the peripheral blood, 24 hours after exposure (Mamedov, 1979).

Groups of 20 male Wistar rats (weight 160–210 g) were exposed to isoprene vapour at concentrations of 27.6 to 100.9 mg/l air for 4 hours. In the same way, groups of 20 female Wistar rats were exposed to vapour concentrations of 29.5 to 98.1 mg/l air. The LC_{50} values were determined as >100.9 mg/l air for the males, and >98.1 mg/l air for the females. The only symptom of toxicity was general malaise in the rats exposed to the highest concentration (Kimmerle and Solmecke, 1972).

Groups of 20 male NMRI mice (weight 18–22 g) were exposed to isoprene vapour at concentrations of 14.1 or 31.5 mg/l air for 4 hours. An LC_{50} value of >31.5 mg/l air was determined. Symptoms of toxicity were comparable to those in the rat (Kimmerle and Solmecke, 1972).

Rabbits exposed for 40 minutes to 4.1 mg/l ($\overset{\wedge}{=}$1470 ppm, n=6) showed a diminished but quicker-acting flexor reflex. The respiratory rate was increased by between 16.3 and 40% at a concentration of about 0.19 mg/l ($\overset{\wedge}{=}$68 ppm) or more (Gostinskii, 1965).

Groups of 30 male Wistar rats were investigated for the cumulative effect of isoprene in a modified Lim-Test (Lim et al., Arch. Int. Pharmacodyn., 130, 336 (1961)). In this study, a dose of 200 mg/kg was administered orally to 30 rats on the first day of the study, and the dose was increased by a factor of 1.5 on the following 4 days. The observation period ended one week after the last dose. This study did not demonstrate any cumulative effect of isoprene in male rats (Kimmerle and Solmecke, 1972).

Groups of ten male and ten female Wistar rats (weight 160–210 g) were exposed to isoprene vapour for 4 hours daily for 5 days at concentrations of 12.7 or 57.3 mg/l air. Both sexes tolerated the highest concentration without effect (Kimmerle and Solmecke, 1972).

An inhalation exposure study was carried out for 2 weeks in F-344 rats and B6C3F1 mice with isoprene at concentrations of 0, 438, 875, 1650, 3500 and 7000 ppm. While the 2-week inhalation exposure was tolerated without symptoms in the rat, the mice showed haematological changes in the form of aplastic anaemia, and histopathological examination revealed testicular atrophy, degeneration of the olfactory epithelium and hyperplasia of the forestomach epithelium (Melnick et al., 1988).

Wistar mice were exposed to 0.098±0.004 mg isoprene/l air ($\hat{=}$35.1±1.6 ppm) or 1.016±0.028 mg/l ($\hat{=}$364±10.0 ppm) by inhalation for 4 hours/day over 30 days. Investigations on days 2, 4, 8, 15 and 30 of the study included determinations of the spleen and thymus weights, the number of cells and mitotic index in the thymus, and the number of lymphocytes in the peripheral blood. No further information was given on the number of animals per group or the type of control group, amongst other things. During exposure, there was a phasic decrease in the number of cells in the thymus in both dose groups, as well as a significant inhibition of mitosis ($p \leq 0.02$), significantly increased lymphocyte levels in the peripheral blood ($p \leq 0.05$), a decreased thymus weight and a significant increase in the weight of the spleen ($p \leq 0.001$). After 30 days of exposure, the mitotic index in the thymus was increased in the low-dose group, while in the high-dose group both the number of cells and the mitotic index were significantly reduced ($p \leq 0.02$ and $p \leq 0.05$, respectively; Mamedov, 1979).

7.3 Skin and mucous membrane effects

Isoprene can penetrate the intact skin of mice, rats and rabbits, and leads to local irritation (no further details, Gostinskii, 1965).

Isoprene is irritating to the eyes (no further details; Mamedov, 1979).

Two New Zealand white rabbits (weight 2.8 to 3.8 kg) each had one ear brushed twice a day with isoprene on 5 consecutive days. Only a transient reddening of the skin occurred, which was regarded by the authors as a low grade skin-damaging effect (Kimmerle and Solmecke, 1972).

7.4 Sensitization

No information available

7.5 Subchronic and chronic toxicity

Wistar mice were exposed to isoprene concentrations of 0.0108±0.00015 mg/l ($\hat{=}$3.9±0.05 ppm) or 0.116±0.0017 mg/l ($\hat{=}$41.6±0.6 ppm) for 4 hours daily, five days a week over 4 months. The mice were assessed as in the aforementioned subacute study after 1, 2, 3, 4 and 5 months, where the 5th month served as an observation period. No information was given on the number of animals per group or the type of control group. In the low-dose group no effects were seen during exposure, but the mitotic index in the thymus was significantly increased ($p \leq 0.01$) at the end of the one-month observation period. In the high-dose group, a significant decrease ($p \leq 0.001$) or increase ($p \leq 0.01$) in the number of thymus cells occurred phasically, which progressed to a significantly decreased ($p \leq 0.01$) or increased ($p \leq 0.02$) thymus weight. The mitotic index of the thymus was significantly reduced ($p \leq 0.001$) throughout the exposure period. All values returned to normal during the one-month observation period (Mamedov, 1979).

Thirty-six mice, eleven rats and five rabbits were exposed to isoprene for 4 hours/day by inhalation. The isoprene concentration in the inhalation chamber varied between 2.2 and 4.9 mg/l air ($\stackrel{\wedge}{=}$789 to 1756 ppm). The mice and rabbits were exposed for 4 months, the rats for 5 months. No details were given on the number of animals of each species in the control group. No influence on the behaviour or body weight gain of the mice was seen during the investigation. A neuropharmacological assessment at the end of the study revealed an impaired performance in the swimming test (16.1 minutes, control 33.9 minutes). In the rat, decreased oxygen consumption was recorded from the third month of treatment, with values of 2210 and 1860 ml/hour/kg body weight for the control and treated groups, respectively. In rabbits, increased leukocyte and slightly decreased erythrocyte levels were seen; the haemoglobin content remained unaffected. At autopsy, increased lung, kidney and brain weights were recorded in all of the surviving animals. Histopathological examination revealed the following findings:

Mouse: degenerative changes in the liver.

Rat/rabbit: Irritation of the bronchi and damage to the lungs (increase in goblet cells in the bronchial mucosa, infiltration of the bronchial walls by inflammatory cells, damage of epithelial cells of the bronchi, vasculitis with perivascular oedema), irritation of the thyroid gland (rat), damage to the myocardium in rabbits (interstitial infiltration, loss of cross-striation). No further details of the study protocol or its findings are given in the publication (Gostinskii, 1965).

Rats exposed to 70–210 ppm isoprene for 6 hours daily over 6 months (no further details) formed reduced quantities of hippuric acid in the liver. Histopathological examination revealed bronchitis, hyperplasia of the lymph nodes in the lungs and histocytic infiltration of the liver and heart (Korbakova and Fedorova, 1964).

7.6   Genotoxicity

7.6.1 In vitro

The mutagenic properties of isoprene were studied in *Salmonella typhimurium* strains TA 98, TA 100, TA 1535 and TA 1537.

In this investigation concentrations of 100, 333, 1000, 3333, and 10,000 µg/plate were used; dimethylsulphoxide was employed as a solvent. Isoprene was cytotoxic at the highest concentration. The tests were carried out with and without metabolic activation (S9 from Aroclor 1254-induced rat or Syrian hamster liver). There were no indications of mutagenicity (Mortelmans et al., 1986).

Similarly, no evidence of mutagenic activity was found in a further study on *Salmonella typhimurium* strains TA 98, TA 100, TA 1530, TA 1535 and TA 1538 with and without metabolic activation (S9 from Aroclor-induced rat liver). Atmospheric concentrations of 25% v/v (up to 75% v/v for strain TA 1538) were tested. The exposure time was 24 hours (DeMeester et al., 1981).

In two further studies on *Salmonella typhimurium* – strains TA 102 and TA 104 were used in the study of Kushi et al. – no mutagenic activity was seen (nor further details; NTP, 1983; Kushi et al., 1985).

The following isoprene metabolites were investigated (without metabolic activation) for mutagenic activity in *Salmonella typhimurium* strains TA 98 and TA 100. Six plates per concentration were used:

Metabolite	Purity
3,4-Epoxy-3-methyl-1-butene (I)	95%
3,4-Epoxy-2-methyl-1-butene (II)	No information
2-Methyl-1,2,3,4-diepoxybutane (III)	99%

Metabolites (I) and (II) were tested at concentrations of 2 to 300 mM/plate ($\hat{=}$136 to 2043 µg/plate). A cytotoxic effect was seen at the highest concentration. No mutagenic activity was evident for metabolites (I) and (II). Metabolite (III) caused a dose-dependent increase in the number of revertants in both strains, from a concentration of 5 mM/plate ($\hat{=}$341 µg/plate). At this concentration of 5 mM/plate, the number of revertants was 1.5 times greater than control values in strain TA 98, and 2.4 times greater in strain TA 100. At 10 mM/plate ($\hat{=}$681 µg/plate) values were 2.8 and 9.4 times greater and at 15 mM/plate ($\hat{=}$1022 µg/plate) 1.5 and 11.5 times greater than controls in strains TA 98 and TA 100, respectively. Marked alkylating activity was found for metabolite (III) in an in vitro test procedure. Nicotinamide served as a nucleophile. The relative values for metabolites (I), (II) and (III) were 15, 35 and 360, respectively (absolute values not given; Gervasi et al., 1985).

7.6.2 In vivo

Fifteen male mice (no details of strain or age) were exposed to isoprene concentrations of 438, 1750 or 7000 ppm for 6 hours/day over 12 days. A 50 mg bromodeoxyuridine tablet was implanted subcutaneously about one hour before the final exposure. Ten mice per group were killed between 17 and 20 hours after tablet implantation in order to assess chromosomal aberrations. The remaining five mice per group were killed 24 hours after tablet implantation to determine sister chromatid exchange. Colchicine (a spindle poison) was given by intraperitoneal injection to each mouse (2 ml/kg) 2 hours before they were killed. At the same time, a smear of peripheral blood was taken from the tip of the tail of each animal. After killing, the bone marrow was removed and prepared with a special stain (Fluorescence-Immler-technique), while the smear of peripheral blood was stained with acridine orange. The sister chromatid exchange rate, chromosomal aberrations and the mitotic index were determined in the bone marrow cells. Micronucleus formation was assessed in the erythrocytes from the blood smear. The results showed that exposure to isoprene at the concentrations employed caused a significant increase in sister chromatid exchange in the bone marrow cells and increased micronuclei in the peripheral blood. In addition, the average regeneration time of the bone marrow cells was prolonged and there was a reduction in polychromatic erythrocytes in the peripheral blood. The increase in the average regeneration time was only observed in the highest dose group (7000 ppm), while the reduction in erythropoiesis occurred significantly and dose-dependently in all treated groups. In contrast, no signs of chromosomal aberrations were seen. The mitotic index in the bone marrow was not significantly affected (Tice et al., 1988).

7.7 Carcinogenicity

No information available

7.8 Reproductive toxicity

Female Wistar rats received 22, 380 or 1900 mg isoprene/kg body weight/day orally for 4 days (days 9 to 12) during pregnancy. No indications of embryotoxicity or teratogenicity were seen. In the foetuses, a negligible retardation in ossfication of the sternum and, to an even lesser extent, of the occipital bone was found (Tsutsumi et al., 1969).

7.9   Effects on the immune system

Studies indicating an immunological effect are described in detail under 7.2 and 7.5 (Mamedov, 1979).

In further studies on rabbits (strain, age and weight not given) which were exposed to 400 mg isoprene/m^3 air for up to 4 months, a decrease in the number of phagocytes was seen (no further details; Faustov, 1972).

Rabbits exposed to 135 ppm isoprene vapour for 4 hours/day over 4 months showed a decrease in isoenzymes, nucleic acids and proteins in the blood serum. In addition, a decrease in phagocytic activity was seen (no further details; Samedov et al., 1971).

Rabbits which were exposed to isoprene vapour (concentrations not given) for 4 hours daily over 2 months showed a decrease in total proteins and an increase in the albumin-globulin ratio in the bone marrow (no further details; Faustov and Lobeeva, 1970).

7.10 Neurotoxicity

No information available

7.11 Other effects

The results already described under 7.6 indicate a cytotoxic effect for isoprene in bone marrow cells (increasing their average regeneration time) and a dose-dependent decrease in polychromatic erythrocytes (inhibiting erythropoiesis in the peripheral blood; Tice et al., 1988).

8.   Experience in humans

One woman and two men were each exposed to various concentrations of isoprene for 5 minutes to determine the odour threshold. The following results were seen: 0.278 mg/l just perceptible; 0.695 mg/l clearly perceptible; 2.78 mg/l very clearly perceptible; 13.9 mg/l very clearly perceptible, headache; 27.8 mg/l clear bronchial irritation, severe headache (Kimmerle and Solmecke, 1972).

Concentrations of 0.16 mg/l air ($\hat{=}$57.4 ppm) and above caused slight irritation of the mucous membranes of the nose, larynx and pharynx in volunteers (n=10). The odour threshold was 0.01 ml/l ($\hat{=}$3.6 ppm; Gostinskii, 1965).

According to Muir (1977) liquid isoprene is also irritating to the skin and eyes.

Inhalation exposure to gaseous isoprene over a long period (no further details) led to a decrease in the number of phagocytes and the phagocytic index in workers at rubber factories. The number of phagocytes decreased to 51–54% of the normal level for periods of employment of up to 5 years, and to about 30% for 15–19 years. Irritation of the upper respiratory tract, influenza, angina and liver and biliary diseases were found to increase with increasing duration of exposure (Faustov, 1972).

Drop tests on the skin of workers in rubber factories produced marked effects after 2–3 months. Itching of the face, forearms and backs of the hands were observed, followed by dermatitis and eczema. The skin appeared dry and flaky on prolonged exposure. A positive reaction was seen in at least 10% of the treated workers (Pigolev, 1971).

The proportion of isoprene in the hydrocarbons excreted in exhaled air was between 30 and 70% (Gelmont et al., 1981).

In the investigations of DeMaster and Gelmont, no distinctions were made with regard to sex, age, racial origin, type of diet, life-style or fasted or unfasted state of the volunteers. The isoprene values were higher during the night. (see table 11).

Table 11. Amounts of isoprene measured in exhaled air

	Isoprene content
30 volunteers	2–4 mg/24 hours ≙ 83–167 µg/hour ≙ 0.19–0.38 µg/l breath[a] (Gelmont et al., 1981)
8 volunteers 5 non-smokers	16–250 µg/hour ≙ 0.04–0.56 µg/l breath[a]
3 smokers	15–390 µg/hour ≙ 0.03–0.88 µg/l breath[a] (Conkle, 1975)
25 volunteers (period of determination 8.00–20.00 hours)	28.3 ± 9.7 nmol/l alveolar air (DeMaster et al., 1976)

[a] At an assumed respiratory volume of 7.4 l/minute

Table 12. Distribution of isoprene and its metabolites after inhalation exposure of male rats[a] to 1480 ppm isoprene for 6 hours (Dahl et al., 1987)

Provisionally characterized metabolites	Freezing point (°C)	nmol/total tissue (at the end of exposure)					
		Nasal cavity	Lungs	Liver	Kidneys	Fat	Blood
Isoprene	−130	44.5	n.d.	0.08	9.91	566	5.10
3,4-Epoxy-3-methyl-1-butene	− 95	3.99	0.24	0.50	4.55	72.4	3.90
3,4-Epoxy-2-methyl-1-butene	− 95						
trans-3-Methyl-1-butene-3,4-diol	− 45						
trans-2-Methyl-1-butene-3,4-diol	− 45	27.6	27.1	235	64.7	2890	230
2-Methyl-1,2,3,4-diepoxybutane	− 45						
Conjugate tetrole	Not volatile	737	391	5520	1500	37770	5590
CO_2[b]	−196	2.77	1.07	15.6	12.6	597	201

n.d. not detected
[a] 4 animals were exposed
[b] Determined exclusively as radioactively-labelled CO_2.

Table 13. Concentration of isoprene and its metabolites in the blood at the end of exposure of male rats[a] to isoprene (Dahl et al., 1987)

Provisionally characterized metabolites	Freezing point °C	^{14}C equivalents in the blood (nmol/animal)			
		8 ppm for 6 hours	260 ppm for 6 hours	1480 ppm for 6 hours	8200 ppm for 5.5 hours
Isoprene	−130	n.d.	n.d.	5.1	384
3,4-Epoxy-3-methyl-1-butene	− 95	n.d.	n.d.	3.9	65
3,4-Epoxy-2-methyl-1-butene	− 95				
trans-3-Methyl-1-butene-3,4-diol	− 45				
trans-2-Methyl-1-butene-3,4-diol	− 45	5.6	110	230	257
2-Methyl-1,2,3,4-diepoxybutane	− 45				
Conjugate, tetrole	Not volatile	90.8	2230	5590	5530
CO_2[b]	−196	0.5	10.9	201	96

n.d. not detected
[a] 4 animals/group were exposed
[b] determined exclusively as radioactively-labelled CO_2

Conkle et al. (1975) postulated that stress, kind of diet, activity and the environment could influence the level of isoprene in the breath.

The activity of various enzyme systems (succinate dehydrogenase, acid and alkaline phosphatase) was assessed in workers at rubber factories. While succinate dehydrogenase activity was suppressed, both acid and alkaline phosphatase activities were increased (Mamedov and Aliev, 1985 a, b).

However, it should be noted that exposure to styrene, butadiene and chloromethane occurred simultaneously and the findings cannot be unequivocally attributed to isoprene. The wearing of rubber gloves (which contain isoprene, amongst other substances) may have led to absorptive effects on the skin as well as sensitization and general toxicity (no further details; Es'kova-Szkovets et al., 1986).

9.   Threshold limit values

A MAK-value of 0.04 mg/l air has been recommended in the Soviet Union (Shugaev, 1969).

References

Clayton, G.D., Clayton, F.E. (eds.)
Patty's Industrial Hygiene and Toxicology
John Wiley, New York, volume 2B, 3196–3220 (1982)

Conkle, J.P., Camp, B.J., Welch, B.E.
Trace composition of human respiratory gas
Arch. Environ. Health, 30, 290–295 (1975)

Dahl, A.R., Birnbaum, L.S., Bond, J.A., Gervasi, P.G.,
Henderson, R.F.
The fate of isoprene inhaled by rats: Comparison to butadiene
Toxicol. Appl. Pharmacol., 89, 237–248 (1987)

Del Monte, M., Citti, L., Gervasi, P.G.
Isoprene metabolism by liver microsomal monooxygenases
Xenobiotica, 15, 591–597 (1985)

DeMaster, E.G., Alexander, C.S., Nagasawa, H.T.
Isoprene, an endogenous constituent of human alveolar air.
Appearance of a diurnal rhythm
Fed. Proc., 35, 838 (1976)

De Meester, C., Mercier, M., Poncelet, F.
Mutagenic activity of butadiene, hexachlorobutadiene and isoprene
In: Industrial and Environmental Xenobiotics
Editors: I. Gut, M. Cikrt and G.L. Plaa
Springer, Berlin Heidelberg New York, 195–203 (1981)

Egle, J.L., Gochberg, B.J.
Retention of inhaled isoprene and methanol in the dog
Am. Ind. Hyg. Assoc. J., 36, 369–373 (1975)

Es'kova-Szkovets, K.B., Bol'schakov, A.M., Vorob'eva, S.N., Tarazin, V.V.
Hygienic assessment of rubber goods made of aryl-polymers
Gig. Sanit., 1, 12–14 (1986)

Faustov, A.S.
The toxic-hygienic characteristics of the gas factor in production of several types of common synthetic rubber
Trudy Voronezhskii Meditsinskii Institut, 87, 10–16 (1972)

Faustov, A.S., Lobeeva, N.V.
Action of some chemical substances on the protein content of serum and bone marrow
Chemical Abstracts, 73, 118648C (1970)

Gelmont, D., Stein, R.A., Mead, J.F.
Isoprene – the main hydrocarbon in human breath
Biochem. Biophys. Res. Commun., 99, 1456–1460 (1981)

Gervasi, P.G., Citti, L., Del Monte, M., Longo, V., Benetti, D.
Mutagenicity and chemical reactivity of epoxidic intermediates of the isoprene metabolism and other structrurally related compounds
Mutat. Res., 156, 77–82 (1985)

Gostinskii, V.D.
Toxicity of isoprene and maximal safe concentration of the vapour in air
Fed. Prod. (trans. suppl.), 24, 1123–1126 (1965)
See also: Gostinskii, V.D.
The toxicity of isoprene and the maximum permissible concentration of its vapours in the atmosphere of industrial premises
Gig. Tr. Prof. Zabol., 9, 36–42 (1965)

Kimmerle, G., Solmecke, B.
Isopren – Akute Toxizitätsuntersuchungen
Bayer AG, unpublished report No. 3373 (1972)

Korbakova, A.J., Fedorova, V.S.
Toxicology of isoprene
Toksikol. Novykk. Prom. Khim. Veshchesto., 6, 18–29 (1964)

Kushi, A., Yoshida, D., Mizusaki, S.
Mutagenicity of gaseous nitrogen oxides and olefins on Salmonella
TA 102 and TA 104
Mutat. Res., 147, 263–264 (1985)

Longo, V., Citti, L., Gervasi, P.G.
Hepatic microsomal metabolism of isoprene in various rodents
Toxicol. Lett., 29, 33–37 (1985)

Lyman, W.J., Rickl, W.F., Rosenblatt, D.H. (eds.)
Handbook of Chemical Property Estimation Methods
McGraw-Hill, New York (1982)

Mamedov, A.M.
Response of lymphoid tissue to single and multiple inhalation expo-
sures to isoprene and some relevant integral indices
Gig. Tr. Prof. Zabol., 34–37 (1979)

Mamedov, A.M., Aliev, V.A.
Succinate dehydrogenase activity of immunocompetent cells in
workers with occupational exposure in styrene and butadiene rubber
production
Azerb. Med. Zh., 62, 25–29 (1985a)

Mamedov, A.M., Aliev, V.A.
Activity of acid and alkaline phosphatases of blood neutrophiles in
workers engaged in the manufacture of synthetic rubber
Gig. Tr. Prof. Zabol., 5, 31–35 (1985b)

Melnick, R., Royeroft, J., Chou, B., Ragan, H., Miller, R.
Inhalation toxicology of isoprene in F 344 rats and B6C3F1 mice
International Symposium on the toxicology, carcinogenesis and
human health aspects of 1,3-butadiene
NIEHS, Research Triangle Park, N.C., USA (1988)

Mortelmans, K., Haworth, S., Lawlor, T., Speck, W., Tainer, B., Zeiger, E.
Salmonella mutagenicity tests: II. Results from the testing of 270 chemicals
Environ. Mutagen., 8 (7), 1–119 (1986)

Muir, G.D. (ed.)
Hazards in the chemical laboratory, 2nd ed., p. 16
The Chemical Society, London (1977)

NTP (National Toxicology Program)
Salmonella mutagenesis test results
NTP, Tech. Bull., 9, 5–6 (1983)

Peter, H., Wiegand, H.J., Bolt, H.M., Greim, H., Walter, G., Berg, M., Filser, J.G.
Pharmacokinetics of isoprene in mice and rats
Toxicol. Lett., 36, 9–14 (1987)

Pigolev, S.A.
Occupational diseases of the skin of workers under conditions of isoprene rubber production
Vestnik Dermatologii i Venerologii, 2, 64–65 (1971)

Samedov, J.G., Mamedov, A.M., Mamedova, L.N., Bekeshev, J.A.
Immunological indices as possible criteria for the judgements on the effects of low-intensity chemical factor on the body
Azerb. Med. Zh., 55, 58–61 (1971)

Shugaev, B.B.
Distribution in the organism and toxicity of aliphatic hydrocarbons
Farmakol. Toksikol., 31, 162–165 (1968)

Shugaev, B.B.
Concentrations of hydrocarbons in tissues as a measure of toxicity
Arch. Environ. Health, 18, 878–882 (1969)

Stahl, W.H. (ed.)
Compilation of odor and taste threshold value data
American Society for Testing and Materials, Philadelphia (1973)
Cited in: Clayton G.D., Clayton F.E., (1982)

Tice, R.R., Boucher, R., Luke, C.A., Paquette, D.E., Melnick, R.C., Shelby, M.D.
Chloroprene and isoprene: cytogenetic studies in mice
Mutagen., 3, 141–146 (1988)

Tsutsumi, S., Yamaguchi, T., Komatsu, S., Tamura, S.
On the teratogenic effects of vitamin A – like substances
Proc. Congenital Anomalies Res. Assoc., Ann. Rep. No. 9, 27 (1969)

Weitz, H.M., Schwarz, H.
Isopren In: Ullmanns Enzyklopädie der technischen Chemie
4th edition, Volume 13, 379–88
Verlag Chemie, Weinheim (1975)

Acrylic acid

The available literature up until 1981 on the toxicity of acrylic acid has been summarized in the "Toxikologisch-arbeitsmedizinischen Begründung" produced by the Commission for the Investigation of Health Hazards of Chemical Compounds in the Work Area, under the auspices of the Deutsche Forschungsgemeinschaft (German Research Association). As a number of additional toxicological studies have become known since then, BG Chemie has compiled the present Toxicological Evaluation. The data contained in the MAK "Begründungen" have been incorporated in the appropriate sections of the Toxicological Evaluation.

1.   Summary and assessment

Radiolabelled acrylic acid is rapidly absorbed through the gastro-intestinal tract and the lungs, and radioactive carbon dioxide is respired just 15 minutes after oral administration. Within 24 hours, 50 to 75% of the acrylic acid is eliminated, 44 to 68% being exhaled as carbon dioxide with the excretion of a further amount via the urine and the faeces. 19 to 25% of the radioactivity is still present in the tissues after 72 hours. In addition to unchanged acrylic acid, 3-hydroxypropionic acid and two unidentified metabolites are found in the urine. The detection of hydroxypropionic acid suggests that acrylic acid is involved in propionic acid and fatty acid metabolism. There are no indications of epoxidation of acrylic acid.

Acrylic acid is of moderate acute toxicity by oral, dermal or inhalation exposure [rat oral LD_{50} 193 to 3200 mg/kg; rabbit dermal LD_{50} 295 to approx. 950 mg/kg; rat LC_{50}, 4 hours 3600 mg/m^3 (1200 ppm)]. Local irritant or corrosive action is the main symptom of intoxication. A single oral dose of acrylic acid causes haemorrhage and oedema in the stomach, accompanied by a non-protein sulphhydryl depletion. The wide spread of the LD_{50} values observed with oral application may be attributed to the different forms in which the acrylic acid is applied (undiluted, or in aqueous, or neutralized solution).

After repeated oral dosing with acrylic acid at locally tolerated concentrations there is decreased intake of food and water, and slower weight increase. Higher concentrations of acrylic acid cause irritation and ulceration of the stomach, the extent being dependent on dose and concentration. Other effects include pulmonary oedema/emphysema and kidney lesions (tubular necrosis) with corresponding changes in the relevant blood parameters (increased levels of glucose, urea nitrogen, and alkaline phosphatase) and urinary parameters (increased levels of protein and increased specific densities). The weights of various organs are decreased, but pathological and histological investigation does not reveal any organ lesions, other than the aforementioned changes in the gastro-intestinal tract and the kidneys. Clinical-chemical and blood parameters do not indicate any pathological changes with the exception of those mentioned above. Repeated oral administration of locally-tolerated acrylic acid concentrations results in a no-effect level of less than 83 mg/kg. Repeated inhalation exposure causes irritation of the nasal mucosa (mainly the olfactory epithelium) and slight hyperplasia of the submucosal glands. These changes are observed in rats and, to a greater extent, in mice (down to 5 ppm). Repeated dermal application results in degenerative and inflammatory changes of the epidermis and dermis.

Acrylic acid is acutely corosive to the skin and eyes.

In itself, acrylic acid is not sensitizing; however, industrial acrylic acid may contain varying amounts of α,β-diacryloxypropionic acid, the presence of which can apparently account for the sensitizing action of industrial acrylic acid, as observed in various animal tests. Distilled acrylic acid does not contain α,β-diacryloxypropionic acid.

After longer-term administration, characteristic systemic lesions of the internal organs (assessed for functional and anatomic as well as histopathological changes) are not seen by any route of administration, apart from the kidney lesions observed at high oral doses.

In the Salmonella/microsome test, acrylic acid is not mutagenic. It is also negative in the HGPRT test, as well as in two UDS tests. In CHO cells and mouse lymphoma cells, acrylic acid causes dose-dependent chromosomal aberrations, but not so in 4 CHL cells. A genotoxic effect is observed in the mouse lymphoma test (L5178Y-cells). In SHE cells, acrylic acid does not cause micronucleus-formation or cell transformation. Acrylic acid is not mutagenic in the available in vivo mutagenicity studies (Drosophila test, chromosomal aberrations in the rat). Studies of covalent binding of acrylic acid to

DNA (liver, epidermis) and corresponding investigations in vitro are inconclusive.

No carcinogenic effect is evident after dermal application of acrylic acid or after its administration in the drinking water. A weak carcinogenic effect obtained from a dermal study on mice, which does not meet present-day requirements, does not stand up to critical examination. Furthermore, two local sarcomas observed in mice after subcutaneous application of acrylic acid do not provide conclusive evidence of carcinogenicity.

Abnormalities and malformations (haemangiomas, skeletal malformations) are produced after intraperitoneal administration of undiluted acrylic acid to rats on days 5, 10 and 15 of pregnancy. In a teratogenicity study, inhalation of acrylic acid, did not cause embryotoxic or teratogenic effects, even at maternally toxic doses. After injection into the amniotic sac on day 13 of pregnancy, acrylic acid is slightly embryotoxic (resorptions only occurring at a dose of 1000 µg/foetus), but there is no evidence of teratogenicity. The reproductive toxicity of acrylic acid in a single-generation study is low, even at doses which harm the parents.

The injuries described in humans are due to the strongly corrosive and blistering action of acrylic acid and acrylic acid vapours or aerosols. Severe, painful injuries to the skin, eyes and the respiratory tract are described. There are no indications of a sensitizing effect in humans. In patients who have shown a hypersensitive reaction to acrylate- or methacrylate-based sealing compounds, no cross-reaction with acrylic acid is reported.

Acrylic acid and its vapours or aerosols have a corrosive or irritant action on the skin, eyes, respiratory tract and gastro-intestinal tract. Acrylic acid can be absorbed through the skin. The available documents do not indicate that acrylic acid is carcinogenic. The results of investigations of genotoxicity in vitro are incosistent; in vivo tests are negative.

2.   Name of substance

2.1 Usual name	Acrylic acid
2.2 IUPAC-name	Ethene carboxylic acid
2.3 CAS-No.	79-10-7

3.   Synonyms, common and trade names

Ethylene carboxylic acid
2-Propenoic acid
Vinyl carboxylic acid

4.   Structural and molecular formulae

4.1 Structural formula

$$H_2C{=}CH{-}C\overset{\displaystyle O}{\underset{\displaystyle OH}{{<}}}$$

4.2 Molecular formula $C_3H_4O_2$

5.   Physical and chemical properties

5.1 Molecular mass, g/mol	72.06
5.2 Melting point, °C	13–14
5.3 Boiling point, °C	141.6 (at 1010.8 hPa)
5.4 Vapour pressure, hPa	10.3 (at 20 °C) 29.3 (at 40 °C)
5.5 Density, g/cm^3	1.0497 (at 20 °C)
5.6 Solubility in water	fully miscible with water
5.7 Solubility in organic solvents	fully miscible with nearly all organic solvents
5.8 Solubility in fat	no information available
5.9 pH-value	2.13 (72.06 g/l, aqueous solution)
5.10 Conversion factor	1 ppm $\overset{\wedge}{=}$ 2.99 mg/m^3 1 mg/m^3 $\overset{\wedge}{=}$ 0.33 ppm (at 25 °C and 1013 hPa) (Ullmann, 1985; Windholz, 1983; IARC, 1979; Weast, 1979)

6.   Uses

For the manufacture of polymerization products (Ullman, 1985)

7.   Experimental results

7.1 Toxicokinetics and metabolism

After Sprague-Dawley rats were exposed to gaseous [^{11}C]-acrylic acid for 1 minute (head/nose exposure; no clear indication of concentration), 18.3% (SE ± 1.8, n=13) of the radioactivity was found in the muscles of the nose and 28.4% (SE ± 2.8, n=10) in the snout region, 1.5 minutes after the end of exposure. 65 minutes after exposure, there was still 8.1% (SE ± 0.8) in the snout. The radioacitivity measured in the whole head, excluding the snout, was 42.9% (SE ± 3.97, n=10; mucous membranes of nasopharynx, trachea and bones); only low concentrations were measured in the lungs. After 65 minutes, the radioactivity in the liver and fat was significantly higher than after 1.5 minutes; the value was also markedly higher in the stomach. In the authors' opinion, the acrylic acid detected in the upper respiratory tract had been absorbed into the gastro-intestinal tract within 65 minutes. In another study, female Sprague-Dawley rats were given [^{11}C]-acrylic acid as an aqueous solution at a dose of 26 µg/kg by stomach tube. The radioactivity in the various organs were determined after 1, 5, 10, 20, 40 and 65 minutes. According to these investigations, acrylic acid was absorbed rapidly from the stomach. The distribution of radioactivity in the various organs showed an increasing retention between 40 and 60 minutes, especially in the liver, fat and small intestine, and in the brain and kidneys. All together, approx. 37% of the applied dose was retained. Approx. 6% of the radioactivity was excreted via the kidneys within 6 hours. After inhalation exposure and also after administration by stomach tube, 60% of the supplied radioactivity was exhaled as carbon dioxide within 1 hour. The radioactivity in the urine increased during the observation time; after 65 minutes the urine samples contained 1.8%/g (SE ± 0.74, n=5) of the radioactivity from oral administration and 1.9%/g (SE ± 0.4, n=3) of the radioactivity from inhalation exposure. Thus, [^{11}C]-acrylic acid was mainly exhaled via the lungs as radioactive carbon dioxide, and was also partly excreted via the kidneys (Kutzman, 1982).

Three male Sprague-Dawley rats were each given a single dose of 4, 40 and 400 mg/kg [2,3-^{14}C]-acrylic acid in 0.5% aqueous methyl cellulose, by stomach tube. The radioactivity in the urine, faeces and exhaled air was measured. Acrylic acid was absorbed rapidly from the gastro-intestinal tract, radioactive carbon dioxide being detectable in the exhaled air just 15 minutes after administration. Within 8 hours, 35 to 60% of the radioactivity had been eliminated. After 24 hours, 50 to 75% had been eliminated, with 44 to 68% being exhaled as carbon dioxide, and a further proportion excreted via the urine and faeces. After 72 hours, 19 to 25% of the radioactivity could still be detected in various tissues [primarily in fat (11%), muscles (7%) and liver (2%)]. HPLC analysis of the urine revealed [^{14}C]-acrylic acid and, metabolites, 3-hydroxypropionic acid and two compounds which were not further identified. The authors therefore presume that acrylic acid is involved in natural propionic acid metabolism, which might explain the rapid formation of carbon dioxide after administration of acrylic acid. The authors suggested the following metabolic pathway for acrylic acid:

acrylic acid → 3-hydroxypropionic acid

acetyl-SCoA ← $\dot{C}O_2$ ← malonaldehyde acid

2,3-Epoxypropionic acid and N-acetyl-S-(2-carboxy-2-hydroxy-ethyl) cysteine were not detected in the urine, and thus the authors deduced that acrylic acid is not epoxidized to epoxypropionic acid in vivo. This hypothesis is supported by the absence of corresponding metabolites after incubation of [^{14}C]-acrylic acid with rat liver microsomes (DeBethizy et al., 1987).

The dermal penetration capacity of acrylic acid was measured in vitro on excised human skin. The skin (thickness 0.25 mm) was coated with 1 mg of ^{14}C-labelled acrylic acid. Testing was effected in a special system according to E.W. Merrith and E.R. Cooper (Journal Control Release, 1984, 1, 161–162). The vehicles used were phosphate buffer pH 6 or pH 7.4, ethylene glycol and acetone.

According to these investigations, dermal penetration decreased with increasing pH value. The values measured after absorption from ethylene glycol were between those measured with phosphate buffer pH 6 and pH 7.4. Acrylic acid was particularly well absorbed from acetone. The relative penetration flow was estimated on the basis of the cumulative absorption, and the values obtained were 1 for phosphate buffer pH 7, 23 for phosphate buffer pH 6, 15 for ethylene glycol, and >600 for acetone. The decreased penetration capacity with increasing pH was consistent with the decrease in the water/octanol partition coefficient of acrylic acid (D'Souza and Francis, 1988).

In an in vivo experiment by the same authors, male Sprague-Dawley rats (weight 200 to 220 g) were administered 50 mg ^{14}C-labelled acrylic acid/kg body weight, dermally. Phosphate buffer pH 6 and pH 7.4 or acetone were used as formulating agents. In each case the formulation was applied to the shaved back of the rats and covered with a glass chamber. The urine and faeces were collected cumulatively (24 hours); carbon dioxide was measured 0.5, 1, 2, 4, 8, 16 and 24 hours after application. The rats were killed after 24 hours, and the levels of radioactivity were determined in the urine, faeces, body tissues, skin and in the exhaled carbon dioxide. The level of radiolabelled carbon dioxide in the respired air was a measure of the absorption of ^{14}C-labelled acrylic acid. The results of the in vivo investigations were comparable to those of the in vitro studies. The absorption rate of the acrylic acid in the different vehicles decreased from acetone > phosphate buffer pH 6.0 > phosphate buffer pH 7.4 (D'Souza and Francis, 1988).

The penetration of ^{14}C-acrylic acid was tested in another in vitro investigation on human and mouse skin. For this purpose, human and mouse skin were treated in a diffusion chamber with the following concentrations of acrylic acid: 0.01, 0.1 and 4% acetone, water or phosphate buffer (pH 6.5). For measurement of absorption, samples were taken between 0 and 32 hours. According to these investigations the rates of absorption of acrylic acid depended on the vehicle; they increased in the order phosphate buffer (pH 6.5), water, acetone. Independently of the vehicle, the absorption rate also increased as a function of the acrylic acid concentration. Mouse skin proved to be three times more permeable than human skin, though the authors did not regard this as a biologically significant difference. The concentration of acrylic acid in the skin (measured after application of 1% preparations) was highest, both for human and mouse skin, after application of acrylic acid in acetone (ICI, 1988).

7.2 Acute and subacute toxicity

The results of acute toxicity studies are shown in the following table:

Table 1. LD_{50}/LC_{50} values for acrylic acid

Species	Route of application	LD_{50}/LC_{50} (mg/kg), (mg/m^3)	Remarks	References
Mouse	oral	240		Boyland, 1940
Mouse	oral	1200		BASF, 1958
Mouse	oral	830		Klimkina, 1969
Mouse	i.p.	140		BASF, 1958
Mouse	i.p.	128 (LDlo)		Nat. Res. Council, 1951
Rat	i.p.	22–24		Majka, 1974 Singh, 1972
Rat	oral	193	anhydrous acrylic acid	Union Carbide, 1977
Rat	oral	340	anhydrous acrylic acid	Carpenter, 1974
Rat	oral	1350		Majka, 1974
Rat	oral	1500		BASF, 1978
Rat	oral	2520		Patty, 1967
Rat	oral	2500		Smyth, 1962
Rat	oral	2100–3200		Miller, 1964, cited in IARC, 1979
Rat	oral	1250		Klimkina, 1969
Rat	inhalation (4 hours)	3600 (1200 ppm)		Majka, 1974
Rat	inhalation (4 hours)	> 5100 (>1740 ppm)		BASF, 1980

Table 1 (continued)

Species	Route of application	LD_{50}/LC_{50} (mg/kg), (mg/m^3)	Remarks	References
Rat	inhalation (5 hours)	LClo 19 g/m^3 (approx. 6000 ppm)		Gage, 1970
Rat	inhalation (3.5 hours)	saturated atmosphere		Clayton and Clayton, 1982
Rat	inhalation (8 hours)	saturated atmosphere	no deaths	Smyth, 1962
Rat	inhalation (4 hours)	LC$_0$ 11.5 g/m^3 (approx. 4000 ppm)	no deaths	Clayton and Clayton, 1982
Rat	inhalation (4 hours)	2000 ppm	0/6 rats	Carpenter, 1974
Rat	inhalation (1 hour)	saturated atmospheres	no deaths	Carpenter, 1974
Rat	inhalation	atmosphere with maximum possible enrichment		BASF, 1979a
	30 minutes		0/12	
	1 hour		1/6	
	3 hours		6/6	
Rat	inhalation (1 hour)	1442 and 1394 ppm (static) 2352 ppm (dynamic)	no deaths Irritation: eye, nose; weight reduction over 8 days	Nachreiner, 1988
Rabbit	oral	250		Klimkina, 1969
Rabbit	dermal	approx. 950		Patty, 1967

Table 1 (continued)

Species	Route of application	LD_{50}/LC_{50} (mg/kg), (mg/m^3)	Remarks	References
Rabbit	dermal	750		Union Carbide, 1977
Rabbit	dermal	295		Carpenter, 1977
Rabbit	dermal	approx. 640		BASF, 1979b

The oral LD_{50} values in rats and mice varied considerably (rat LD_{50} between 193 and 3200 mg/kg, mouse LD_{50} between 830 and 2400 mg/kg). As far as it is possible to tell from the information provided, this wide variation can be explained by the different forms in which the acrylic acid was applied i.e. undiluted, in aqueous solution at various concentrations, or in neutralized solution.

One hour after oral administration of acrylic acid at concentrations of 0.08, 0.8, 8 or 20% w/v in 0.5% aqueous methyl cellulose (corresponding to doses of 4, 40, 400 and 1000 mg/kg), there was a considerable increase in weight of the stomach and forestomach at doses of >0.8% acrylic acid, which was accompanied by pronounced oedema and haemorrhage. Pre-treatment with the carboxyl esterase inhibitor TOCP (tri-o-cresylphosphate), did not produce any significant changes compared with the results obtained without TOCP pre-treatment (DeBethizy et al., 1987).

When male Holtzmann rats (240 to 300 g) were exposed to concentrations of 100, 300 and 500 ppm for 1 hour, there were decreases in the respiratory rate, minute volume and rectal temperature as a function of the severity of local irritation in the respiratory tract (investigations on 5 animals in each case; Silver et al., 1981).

Male F-344 rats received a single dose of acrylic acid by stomach tube at a dose of 144 mg/kg in corn oil (2 mmol/5 ml corn oil/kg). Four hours after dosing, superficial necrosis of the stomach was seen in two out of seven rats. After changing the solvent (water plus Emulphor), extending the follow-up period (24 hours) or even increasing the dose [290 mg/kg (4 mmol/5 ml corn oil/kg)], the local

irritant effect did not become more pronounced (gravimetric measurement of stomach oedema; Ghanayem et al., 1985).

The acute toxicity of acrylic acid after oral, parenteral, dermal and inhalation exposure was relatively low. The main symptoms of intoxication were local irritant and corrosive effects, and general, non-characteristic symptoms (e.g. prostration, tremor, dyspnoea). After single application, the macroscopic changes found at autopsy were in accordance with the irritant properties of acrylic acid.

Motor excitation and spasms were observed after intraperitoneal administration. Dermal application resulted in dyspnoea, diarrhoea and blood in the urine. Inhalation exposure was followed by eye irritation with damage to the cornea, respiratory tract irritation, dyspnoea and pulmonary oedema and, at high concentrations, skin lesions (LC_{50} approx. 1200 ppm).

Five male and five female F-344 rats received acrylic acid in the drinking water at concentrations of 0.6, 0.3 or 0.15% (males approx. 0.68, 0.42 or 0.21 g/kg/day, females 0.76, 0.4 or 0.22 g/kg/day) for 7 days. A significant reduction in weith gain was seen in the high-dose males on days 4 and 7, and a slight reduction (not significant) was seen in high-dose females on day 1. Water intake decreased by 26% in the males and by 19% in the females. Food consumption was unaffected. At both the lower doses, the animals remained unaffected (DePass and Weil, 1983).

Groups of five male and five female F-344 rats (28 days old) and B6C3F1 mice (28 days old) were exposed by inhalation for 6 hours/day for 10 days to 225, 75, 25 or 0 ppm acrylic acid (concentration measured by IR spectrophotometry). At 225 ppm there were signs of nasal irritation (scratching of the nose) in rats and mice. After 4, 7 and 10 days there was a significant reduction in weight-gain of the treated rats and mice, in comparison with the controls. The fat stores in female rats were reduced, but the absolute and relative weights of the organs (brain, heart, liver, kidneys and testes) were unchanged in both species. Histologically, there were inflammatory degenerative lesions of the nasal mucosa, with focal metaplasia. At the lower concentrations of 75 and 25 ppm no clinical signs of nasal irritation were seen in rats and mice. In comparison with the controls, weight gain was unaffected, as were the absolute and relative organ weights. Macroscopically, no clear lesions were observed in the nasal mucosa. Histologically, lesions of the type generally observed with irritant gases were detected in mice exposed to 75 ppm and in some mice exposed to 25 ppm. The distribution of the lesions showed that the olfactory epithelium was more sensitive than the respiratory epithelium (Miller et al., 1981a).

Four male and four female rats (Alderly-Park strain, specifically pathogen-free, weight approx. 200 g) were exposed four times for 6 hours at 1500 ppm. The animals displayed inflammatory changes to the nose, apathy and weight loss; histological investigation revealed congestion in the kidneys. Exposure at 300 ppm (four males and four females exposed 20 times for 6 hours) caused irritation of the nose, apathy, and delayed weight gain. No changes of the internal organs were found at autopsy. A concentration of 80 ppm (four males and four females exposed 20 times for 6 hours) was tolerated without symptoms of intoxication. No organ changes were found at autopsy (Gage, 1970).

Wistar rats (180 to 200 g, number and distribution of sexes not stated) were exposed daily for 4 hours to an acrylic acid concentration of 700 mg/m^3 (238 ppm) for 5 weeks. Weight gain was reduced in comparison with the controls; after 29 and 35 days the excretion of phenol red in the urine (determined after 60 and 120 minutes) was significantly increased ($p < 0.05$ and 0.001). The specific gravity of the urine was significantly lower ($p < 0.05$) in comparison with the controls, and after 30 days the number of reticulocytes was markedly increased ($p < 0.005$). The acrylic acid vapours caused inflammation of the upper respiratory tract and mucosal lesions in the stomach (Majka et al., 1974).

7.3   Skin and mucous membrane effects

In patch tests with undiluted acrylic acid, tissue corrosion was evident within one minute of application to the shaved dorsal skin of white rabbits. After the same exposure time, 50% aqueous solutions led to inflammatory changes with skin reddening and oedema, and 20% solutions still caused slight reddening. After application of a 10% aqueous solution, there were no skin changes even after 15 minutes. All investigations were undertaken using a semi-occlusive method (BASF, 1958).

Undiluted acrylic acid applied to the skin of rabbits for 24 hours caused moderate to severe necrosis (Carpenter et al., 1974).

A 5% acrylic acid solution in acetone caused skin irritation in the mouse (C3H/HeJ strain) after daily open application for 14 days.

A corresponding 1% solution was tolerated without irritation (DePass et al., 1984).

After 1 drop (approx. 50 µl) of undiluted acrylic acid was instilled into the conjunctival sac of the rabbit's eye, there was immediate erosion of the conjunctivae and of the cornea. In the course of 8 to 14 days, complete destruction of the eye occurred (BASF, 1958).

Undiluted acrylic acid applied to the conjunctival sac of the rabbit's eye led to severe eye damage after 18 to 24 hours (Carpenter et al., 1974).

The lowest concentration to cause visible damage to the eye of rabbits was stated to be 1% (Union Carbide, 1977).

7.4   Sensitization

Approx. 0.1 ml of a 20% aqueous solution of acrylic acid (pure acrylic acid, not stabilized) was applied once a day, in the form of a cross, to the shaved left flank of white guinea-pigs, using a cotton swab. This procedure was repeated until definite skin irritation could be seen in the treated region. After an interval of 11 days, a 2% aqueous solution of acrylic acid (ten times weaker, primarily non-irritant) was applied in the same way to the shaved right flank (not previously treated) and the reaction of the skin was recorded after 8, 12 and 24 hours. This study showed that repeated application of a 20% aqueous solution of pure acrylic acid to guinea-pig skin caused degeneration of the tissue with the formation of crusts, the latter being shed and resulting in surface scars. Skin sensitization by repeated application could not be established (BASF, 1958).

In the case of Hartley guinea-pigs (10 animals), 0.1 ml acrylic acid (purity not stated) was applied to the shaved skin of the back, four times in 10 days. After the third application, 0.2 ml of Freund's complete adjuvant was injected intradermally, immediately adjacent to the exposure site. The test substance was applied two weeks after the last application, and the reaction was recorded after 24 and 48 hours. None of the ten guinea-pigs used showed skin sensitization (Rao et al., 1981).

Testing the skin sensitizing efficiency of acrylic acid considering the Polak-method (5 time subcutaneous injection of acrylic acid, purity 99%) in the pad or neck of guinea-pigs, challenge on the flank weekly for 12 weeks (5% acrylic acid solution) resulted in a weak positive reaction at first after 28 days with 3/6 guinea-pigs (Parker and Türk, 1983).

In a further study on guinea-pigs (adjuvant-test) it was be demonstrated that the sensitizing efficiency of technical acrylic acid depends of the presence of α, β-diacryloxypropionic acid as contamination, which is produced obviously during synthesis of acrylic acid. Pure distilled acrylic acid does not content these impurity. None of the guinea-pigs sensitized by technical acrylic acid responded when challenged with the same concentration of acrylic acid purified by distillation (Waagemaekers and van der Walle, 1984).

7.5   Subchronic and chronic toxicity

Young albino rats (Porton strain, no details of number, sex distribution etc.) received sodium acrylate in the diet for 10 weeks at a concentration of 400 mg/kg food, and then for 3 weeks at a concentration of 800 mg/kg food. Four of the rats that had been treated in this way then received a further seven doses of 100 mg/kg in 9 days by stomach tube. Weight increase was unchanged and there were no indications of toxic disturbances of the nervous system (sodium acrylate was investigated in comparison with acrylamide; Barnes, 1970).

Acrylic acid (purity >99%) in distilled water was administered daily by stomach tube five times a week for 3 months, to two groups of ten male and ten female Wistar rats. A control group of ten animals of each sex received distilled water alone. Doses were 150 and 375 mg/kg body weight (application volume 5 ml, corresponding concentrations in distilled water 3 and 7.5%). At the highest dose (375 mg/kg), there was a slight to moderate reduction in growth of the male rats and, to some extent (during the first 3 weeks of testing), of the female rats. Tympan of the gastro-intestinal tract was observed in the majority of the test animals, often associated with cyanosis and dyspnoea, the symptoms starting from the third week of testing. In a few animals an unphysiological sound was stated. Six of the ten male rats and nine of the ten female rats died during the course of the study. Pathological-anatomical and histopathological investigation revealed irritation of the stomach, including thickening of the plica marginata, hyperaemia and bleeding erosions/ulcerations of the gastric mucosa. In addition, there was elevation of the diaphragm, pulmonary oedema/emphysema and alveolar hyperaemia and dystelectases. Catarrhal or catarrhal-suppurative rhinitis was found in some of the animals. In the animals that died during the study, necrotizing tubular nephroses had occurred. In the low-dose group (150 mg/kg), five of the ten males and five of the ten females died during the study. The range of symptoms and the histopathological findings were similar to those seen in the 375 mg/kg group, but were less pronounced and occurred in a smaller number of animals. A no-effect level was not determined (BASF, 1987a).

Groups of 30 male and 30 female rats received acrylic acid (purity >99%) in the drinking water for 3 to 12 months, at concentrations of 5000, 2000, 800, 120 or 0 ppm (corresponding to approx. 375, 150, 60, 10 or 0 mg/kg). Ten males and ten females from each group were killed after 3 months, and the remaining animals after 12 months. After 3 months of treatment, there were no changes in clinical-chemical, haematological or urinary parameters in the four groups, in comparison with controls. Pathological/anatomical and histological examinations confirmed the absence of pathological effects. No changes in organ weights were observed. Reduced intake of water and food, and delayed development of body weight, only occurred in the 5000 and 2000 ppm groups, with the males being affected more than the females. The authors assume a no-effect level between 2000 and 800 ppm (between 150 and 60 mg/kg; BASF, 1987b).

In another subchronic investigation, Fischer-344 rats of both sexes received acrylic acid (purity 99%) for 3 months in the drinking water (no details were given of the concentration), providing a daily intake of approx. 750, 250 and 83 mg/kg [the concentrations in the drinking water must have been between about 10,000 and 1000 ppm (1 and 0.1%)]. Fifteen animals (aged 41 days) of each sex were used per dose group. In the highest dose group (750 mg/kg/day) there was a decrease in the consumption of food and water, and decreases in the body weight and in the absolute weights of the organs (liver, kidneys, spleen, heart, brain, testes). The relative organ weights were higher. There was no change in the numbers of red and white blood cells. Increases were seen in the levels of urea, glucose, alkaline phosphatase and aspartate-transaminase in the blood. Furthermore, in the females there was a statistically significant decrease in serum cholesterol levels. In the urine, there was an increase in the specific gravity and in the protein level. In the females, the pH-value decreased. Comparable though quantitatively smaller effects were measured in the animals of the medium dose group (250 mg/kg). In the low dose group (83 mg/kg), only a reduction in the food and water intake was established. In all groups, there were no macroscopic or microscopic organ changes. The no-effect level was taken to be 83 mg/kg or lower (DePass and Weil, 1980; DePass et al., 1983).

When an aqueous solution of acrylic acid was administered orally to ten mice and ten rats (strain, sex etc. not stated), at a dose of 2.5 mg/kg/day for 3 months, there were changes in the conditioned reflexes. A dose of 0.25 mg/kg administered for the same period no longer caused detectable disturbances of reflexes in rats (Klimkina et al., 1969).

The same authors conducted a six-month study on rabbits (strain, group size etc. not stated) involving administration of acrylic acid at dose levels of 0.025, 0.25 and 2.5 mg/kg/day. The top dose of 2.5 mg/kg resulted in increased chloride values and a lowering of the alkali reserve in the blood, together with degenerative changes in the stomach, intestine, kidneys, adrenal glands, liver, pancreas, spleen and central nervous system. At a dose of 0.25 mg/kg, very few morphological changes were found, and the lowest dose of 0.025 mg/kg no longer produced any detectable effects. The observations are described in detail, but individual findings are not given (Klimkina et al., 1969).

Groups of 30 female mice (aged 42 days) of strains ICR, C3H and B6C3F1 (respective body weights 18.8 to 27.2 g, 22 to 26.5 g and 18.4 to 24.2 g) received dermal applications (dorsally) of acrylic acid in acetone, 3 times per week, for 13 weeks at concentrations of 0, 1 and 4% (application volume 100 µl). Five mice from each group were killed and examined after 1, 2, 4 and 8 weeks, the remainder after 13 weeks. In all three strains of mice, the 4% solution in acetone caused marked skin irritation, desquamation, fissures and crust formation after just 1–2 weeks. These changes became most marked between weeks 3 and 5 and persisted throughout the test. Acetone alone and the 1% acrylic acid solution did not produce any macroscopic changes. Histological investigation revealed proliferative, degenerative and inflammatory changes in the epidermis and dermis in the 4% group after just 1 week, and these changes persisted at about the same level throughout the test period. In the 1% group there were only minimal proliferative changes. No differences in reaction were found between the three strains of mice (Tegeris et al., 1987, 1988).

In a subchronic inhalation study, 3-week-old Fischer-344 rats and B6C3F1 mice of both sexes, were exposed to acrylic acid vapours at concentrations of 0, 5, 25 and 75 ppm for 6 hours/day, 5 days/week for 13 weeks. Fifteen animals of each sex were used, per group. There was no adverse effect on body-weight gain of the rats and mice, with the exception of the female mice exposed to 25 and

75 ppm whose mean body weight was statistically significantly lower at the end of the exposure period. In addition, in comparison with the controls, there was a slight but statistically significant decrease in the hemoglobin level in the male mice exposed to 25 and 75 ppm and in the female mice exposed to 75 ppm. However, the values were within the normal range of variation for this strain and age (historical controls). The organ weights (absolute and relative) were unaffected, and there were no macroscopic changes. Histopathological investigation of the nasal mucosa of ten rats of each sex in the highest dose group (75 ppm), showed slight focal degeneration of the olfactory epithelium in seven out of ten males and ten out of ten females, compared with controls. No such changes were observed in the rats exposed to 25 and 5 ppm. In the mice, histopathological investigation of the nasal mucosa revealed lesions of the olfactory cells in all dose groups. The mice in the highest dose group (75 ppm, all animals investigated) exhibited slight to moderate focal degeneration of the olfactory epithelium with slight cell infiltration and slight hyperplasia of the submucosal glands in the corresponding regions. Replacement of olfactory epithelium by respiratory epithelium was observed in some cases. These effects were dose-dependent, with focal degeneration of the olfactory epithelium seen in ten out of ten males and nine out of ten females in the medium-dose group and in one out of ten males and four out of ten females in the low-dose group. In neither species were any histopathological changes found in the other organs (Miller et al., 1981a).

Different "sensitivities" to the toxic effects of acrylic acid on the nasal mucosa of mice and rats after inhalation exposure for 13 weeks (Miller et al., 1981a, NOEL mice <5 ppm; NOEL rats 25 ppm) can be explained by differences in dosimetry. Acrylic acid is a sensory stimulant and reduces the breathing rate and therefore also the respiratory minute volume (RD_{50} mouse = 513 ppm; RD_{50} rat = 685 ppm; RD_{10} mouse =47 ppm; RD_{10} rat = 48 ppm). After four exposures at 75 ppm, the breathing rate and tidal volume were measured on the fifth day, and a dose ($\mu g/minute/cm^2$) was determined from the calculated respiratory minute volume and the surface area of the nasal mucosa. This is roughly twice as high for the mouse as for the rat, so that the difference in effect might be related more to differences in the amount of active substance, rather than to species-specific sensitivities. The authors recommend that such dosimetric considerations should be taken into account when evaluating species-related differences in reaction to sensory stimulants (Buckley et al., 1984; Barrow, 1987).

7.6   Genotoxicity

7.6.1 In vitro

In the Ames test using Salmonella typhimurium strains TA 1535, TA 1537, TA 98 and TA 100, acrylic acid was tested over a dose range from 3.1 to 1000 nl/plate, with and without S9-mix. In order to increase the sensitivity of the assay, an inhibitor of the enzyme epoxide hydratase was included in some tests, to detect a mutagenic effect by metabolically produced epoxides. Under these conditions, no mutagenic effect could be established for acrylic acid, in contrast to the test substances which were included as controls (N-methyl-N'-nitro-N-nitrosoguanidine, benzo(a)pyrene-4,5-oxide or 2-aminoanthracene,   N-methyl-4-aminostilbene   and   3-methyl-cholanthrene; Oesch, 1977).

Under the same test conditions, and additionally with Salmonella typhimurium strain TA 1538, with and without S9-mix (from rat-liver or hamster-liver homogenate), acrylic acid was not mutagenic over a dose range from 1 to 1000 µg/plate, in contrast to the positive controls   (9-aminoacridine,   2-nitrofluorene,   2-aminoanthracene; Lijinsky and Andrews, 1980).

In another investigation using Salmonella typhimurium strains TA 100, TA 1535, TA 1537 and TA 98, with and without S9-mix (from Aroclor-induced   rat   and   hamster   liver),   acrylic   acid   was   not mutagenic up to concentrations of 1000 µg/plate (Zeiger et al., 1987).

Chinese hamster ovary cells were treated for 4 hours at 37 °C, with and without metabolic activation, with acrylic acid dissolved in distilled water and neutralized to pH 7 with sodium hydroxide. The concentrations were 1615, 2154, 2846 nl/ml (with metabolic acitvation) and 2846, 3769 and 5000 nl/ml (without metabolic activation). Both in the presence and absence of metabolic activation, there was a dose-dependent increase in the number of chromosomal aberrations, except at a dose of 2846 nl/ml without metabolic activation (McCarthy et al., 1988).

Acrylic acid was tested in the HGPRT-assay in vitro, for its ability to induce point-mutations in Chinese hamster ovary cells, in the presence or absence of S9-mix (from Aroclor-induced rat livers). The test concentrations were 0.3, 0.6, 1, 1.5 and 1.9 µl/ml with metabolic activation and 1, 1.5, 1.9, 2.4 and 2.8 µl/ml without metabolic activation. Under these conditions acrylic acid was not mutagenic at any test concentration (Yang, 1988).

The genotoxicity of acrylic acid was also investigated in the mouse lymphoma test (L5178Y cells) without metabolic activation. A dose-dependent increase in the frequency of mutations was observed (at 500 µg/ml, 245 and 325 mutants per 106 surviving cells; controls 61 and 80 mutants per 10^6 surviving cells). There was also a dose-dependent increase in the frequency of chromosomal aberrations in the mouse lymphoma cells (200 µg/ml 7 aberrations, 450 µg/ml 26 aberrations, 500 µg/ml 42 aberrations; Moore et al., 1988).

Conversely, in 4CHL cells (fibroblasts from chinese hamster lung tissue), no chromosomal aberrations were found after addition of acrylic acid at concentrations of 750 µg/ml without metabolic activation (Ishidate et al., 1988).

In a UDS test on primary rat hepatocyte cultures, acrylic acid was negative at concentrations of 0.01, 0.03, 0.06, 0.1, 0.2, 0.3, 0.4 µl/ml (Curren, 1988).

In another UDS test on SHE-cells (Syrian hamster embryo fibroblasts), acrylic acid was again negative (1 to 300 µg/ml). Furthermore, in these cells the numbers of micronuclei were not increased (0.5 to 10.0 µg/ml) and there were no transformations (5 to 50 µg/ml; Wiegand et al., 1989).

Acrylic acid was incubated with various 2-deoxynucleosides (2-deoxyadenosine, 2-deoxycysteine, 2-deoxyguanosine and 2-deoxythymidine) at pH 7 and at 37 °C for 40 days; after this time, 2-carboxyethyl adducts were detected in the preparations. Similar adducts were found on incubation of acrylic acid with the DNA from calf thymus, under the same test conditions. In the opinion of the authors, these adducts were identical to those found with β-propiolactone under the same test conditions. However, the unusually long incubation time of 40 days and the absence of corresponding comparative investigations with a definitely non-carcinogenic organic acid of similar structure and similar molecular weight call into question the relevance of the 2-carboxyethyl adducts found, with regard to the carcinogenic potential of acrylic acid. Nevertheless, on the basis of the adducts found on incubation of acrylic acid with the aforementioned nucleosides, together with the development of 2 sarcomas in 30 female mice [Hsd(ICR)Br-strain] after subcutaneous injection, twice weekly, for 52 weeks (cf. carcinogenicity section, 7.7), the authors concluded that acrylic acid has slight carcinogenic potential (Segal et al., 1987).

In contrast to the investigations of Segal et al., Reynolds and Frederick (1988) found that the incubation of the negatively charged acrylate anion with two representative nucleophiles, methylamine and imidazole, did not result in the formation of adducts of the acrylate ion on the nucleophile. The formation of Michael products in vitro via the non-ionized form of acrylic acid was investigated as an alternative and was found to be theoretically possible, though in the opinion of the authors this is unlikely to occur in vivo because of the rapid metabolism and excretion of acrylic acid.

7.6.2 In vivo

The covalent binding of $[2,3\text{-}^{14}C]$-acrylic acid to liver-DNA from two male rats was investigated 24 hours after a single oral dose (233 and 257 mg/kg respectively). No DNA adducts were found in the liver, nor in the stomach, of these two animals.

To investigate DNA binding of acrylic acid in the epidermis, a 13% or 15% unbuffered solution of $[2,3\text{-}^{14}C]$-acrylic acid in acetone was applied to the shaved skin of female ICR mice (13 and 15 mg/mouse, skin area 8 cm^2). Some animals were pretreated for 7 days with a 5% unlabelled solution of acrylic acid (oedema of the skin). Formation of DNA adducts in the epidermis was detected in both test groups, particularly in the animals which were not pretreated. In view of the discrepancy between these results in mouse skin and the findings obtained in the liver and stomach, the authors consider that further research is needed to elucidate whether the epidermis-DNA-adducts are formed in intact epidermal cells, in damaged epidermal cells with exposed DNA or during DNA isolation (Sagelsdorf et al., 1988).

Acrylic acid was tested for recessive lethal mutations in the Drosophila test using two different routes of administration. In the first test, 2% acrylic acid was given to male Drosophila flies for 3 days as a 5% sucrose solution in their food. No mutagenic effect was produced. To verify the results, acrylic acid at a concentration of 2% was also injected into the abdomen, and again no mutagenic effect of acrylic acid was found in *Drosophila melanogaster* (Valencia et al., 1988).

For analysis of chromosomal changes, male and female Sprague-Dawley rats received a single oral dose of acrylic acid at dose levels of 1000, 330 and 100 mg/kg (dissolved in water, application volume 3 ml/kg). Five animals of each sex per group were killed 6, 12 and 24 hours after dosing. The mitotic index and chromosomal aberrations were determined. No increase in chromosomal aberrations was observed in any of the treated groups in comparison with the controls. The mitotic index of the test groups was also comparable to that of the control group. The effect of repeated administration of acrylic acid on chromosomal aberrations was also determined. Male and female rats received drinking water containing 5000 or 2000 ppm acrylic acid for 5 days. Even after repeated administration, no significant increase in chromosomal aberrations was found, compared with the controls (McCarthy et al., 1988).

7.7 Carcinogenicity

In a carcinogenicity study, three groups each consisting of 50 male and 50 female Wistar rats received acrylic acid in the drinking water at concentrations of 120 ppm (approx. 9 mg/kg), 400 ppm (approx. 31 mg/kg) and 1200 ppm (approx. 88 mg/kg) for 26 months (males) or 28 months (females). The doses and concentrations were derived from the results of a 12-month drinking water study (see Section 7.5). Consumption of drinking water, weight increase, haematological parameters and pathological-anatomical and histological investigation of the organs were recorded. Apart from a marginal reduction in water consumption for both sexes in the highest dose group, there were no toxic changes that could be ascribed to administration of the substance. In particular, there was no indication that acrylic acid was carcinogenic under the conditions of this test (BASF, 1989).

25 µl of a 1% acrylic acid solution in acetone was applied 3 times weekly to the skin of the back of 40 male C3H/HeJ mice throughout their lifetime. Acetone alone was similarly applied to the negative controls, and 0.1% 3-methylcholanthrene was applied to the positive controls. No tumours of the skin or subcutaneous tissue were formed after treatment with acrylic acid or acetone. In the positive control group, 39/40 animals had tumours, 33 of which were malignant epitheliomas. There was no difference in lifespan between the various groups. Acrylic acid was not considered to be carcinogenic. No systemic effects were observed after chronic dermal exposure. Epidermal hyperplasia was seen in one mouse (DePass et al., 1984).

To determine whether acrylic acid acts as a complete carcinogen and/or as a two-stage promoter, acrylic acid in acetone solution (probable dose 4 mg/0.1 ml acetone) was applied 3 times weekly for 1.5 years to the shaved skin of 30 female ICR/Ha mice.

Table 2. Results of the dermal two-stage promoter assay with acrylic acid

1st treatment	2nd treatment	Occurrence of first tumour after x days	Mice with tumours
None	Acrylic acid 4 mg/0.1 ml acetone	361	2 epithelial cell carcinomas (p=0.07)[a]
DMBA 20 μg/ 0.1 ml acetone	Acrylic acid 4 mg/0.1 ml acetone	357	3 papillomas 1 epithelial cell carcinoma (p=0.0035)[b]
DMBA 20 μg/ 0.1 ml acetone	0.1 ml acetone	—	0
None	None	—	0

[a] Relative to historical controls, 1 tumour in 180 animals
[b] Relative to historical controls, 1 tumour in 90 animals

Additional groups were treated with dimethylbenzanthracene and acrylic acid (single dose of 20 μg DMBA/0.1 ml acetonte + 4 mg/ 0.1 ml acrylic acid 3 times weekly), with DMBA alone or were untreated. The results are presented in Table 2. There was no significant difference in number of tumours compared with the controls used in the study. On the basis of these studies, the authors concluded that acrylic acid is a weak complete carcinogen (Cote et al., 1986). Following verification of the individual data, A.D. Little Inc. (1986), concluded that the results of this study are not valid because there is no written study protocol, and the details of the dose of acrylic acid used were different on a presentation poster, in the printed abstract and after further enquiry of the authors (4.0 mg/0.1 ml acetone, 4 mg/0.25 ml acetone, 1 mg/0.1 ml acetone). According to the research by A.D. Little Inc., the dose of acetone used was probably 1 mg/0.1 ml. Furthermore, the results of a pilot study on skin toxicity that had been mentioned were not available. These criticisms are contained in a report by A.D. Little Inc. to the Celanese Corporation (1986). Other investigators (Wiegand et al., 1989) assumed that the local tumours developed as a result of the irritant or corrosive effect of acrylic acid. There was no significant difference (Fischer exact test) between the numbers of tumours in the treated groups and the controls. The significance values given relate to historical controls a) one tumour in 180 animals, b) one tumour in 90 animals. The publication also noted an increased number of leukaemias in the mice treated with acrylic acid in comparison with the historical controls, but this increase did not stand up to critical re-appraisal. There were no detailed histopathological findings for the individual animals. On the basis of the distribution of tumours, it can be assumed with a high degree of probability that the lymphomas observed were not caused by the treatment.

A group of 30 female Hsd: (ICR)Br mice received 20 µmol (1.4 mg) acrylic acid in 0.05 ml trioctanoin subcutaneously (in the left flank), once a week for 52 weeks and were then observed for a further 93 days after the last injection. Corresponding control animals were treated with trioctanoin alone or were untreated. In the mice treated with acrylic acid, 2 sarcomas developed at the application site, the first tumour being observed after 323 days. There were no tumours in the controls (Segal et al., 1987).

With some tumour-promoting substances, it is assumed that there is a positive correlation between tumour-promoting activity and the ability to induce hepatic ornithine-decarboxylase. On the basis of this hypothesis, acrylic acid and a number of food additives were investigated in a larger test series. Male Wistar rats received 0, 0.8, 1.6, 2.4 mg acrylic acid/kg in DMSO by intraperitoneal injection. Acrylic acid did not induce ornithine-decarboxylase, whereas definite signs of induction were found with the comparative products butyl-hydroxyanisole and acrylonitrile (van de Zande et al., 1986).

7.8 Reproductive toxicity

Groups of five female pregnant rats received 0, 2.3, 4.5 or 7.5 µl acrylic acid/kg (1/10, 1/5, 1/3 of LD_{50}), by intraperitoneal injection on days 5, 10 and 15 of pregnancy. The LD_{50} was 22.5 µl/kg. The mothers were killed on day 20 of pregnancy. In all groups, the foetuses of the treated mothers were smaller than those of the control animals ($p < 0.01$). At doses of 4.5 and 7.5 µl/kg, a dose-related increase in haemangiomas was observed in the nape, shoulders, posterior and extremities of the foetuses ($p < 0.05$). At the highest dose, the most frequent abnormalities of the skeletal system were lengthened ribs that were fused with the sternum, deformed rear extremities and missing ribs (p < 0.05). Three of the foetuses were dead. At a dose of 2.3 µl/kg there were no differences in the occurrence of haemangiomas or of skeletal changes compared with the controls. There is no information on maternal toxicity (Singh et al., 1972).

Groups of five pregnant Sprague-Dawley rats were exposed to acrylic acid vapour at concentrations of 0, 25, 75 and 225 ppm, from the 6th to the 15th day post coitum. Observation of the animals continued until the 20th day post coitum, when they were killed. In addition to measuring changes in maternal body weight, intake of feed and water, maternal mortality, and clinical symptoms, anatomical, pathological investigations were undertaken. In the mothers, these included the corpora lutea, uterine and placental weights, number of implantations and ovular loss. In the foetuses, body and organ weights and body length were determined and malformations of the skeleton and of the viscera were assessed. None of the parameters measured showed a significant concentration-dependent change compared with the control group. No signs of prenatal toxicity could be detected under the conditions of this test (BASF, 1981).

Under the same test conditions, but with concentrations of 0, 40, 120 and 360 ppm, there was a reduction in feed and water intake by the mothers exposed at 360 ppm, along with a corresponding decline in body weight gain. The acrylic acid vapours caused irritation of the eyes and respiratory tract, but there were no visceral effects and no evidence of embryotoxicity or teratogenicity (BASF, 1983).

Pregnant Sprague-Dawley rats, anaesthetized with ether, were laparotomized on day 13 of pregnancy. The foetuses in one uterine horn received, acrylic acid in the amniotic sac, at a volume of 10 µl dissolved in 0.9% sodium chloride providing dose levels of 10, 100 or 1000 µg/foetus. The foetuses in the contralateral uterine horn received 10 µl of 0.9% sodium chloride/foetus. The abdominal cavity was then closed up again. The foetuses were investigated on the 20th day of gestation. The doses of 10 and 100 µg acrylic acid/foetus, in comparison with the contralateral controls, did not exhibit any significant foetotoxic effect, whereas a dose of 1000 µg/foetus resulted in the resorption of 78% of the foetuses. Five or six litters were available for each dose. One foetus from the 100 µg group exhibited slight hydrocephalus and micrognathia. No teratogenic effects were observed in the study (Slott and Hales, 1985).

Ten male and 20 female Fischer-344 rats (age 41 to 43 days) received acrylic acid (purity >99%) in the drinking water at doses of 750, 250 and 83 mg/kg/day for 13 weeks. The individual results of these subchronic toxicity investigations are given in Section 7.5. Following this subchronic treatment, the reproductive toxicity was assessed in a single-generation study. Treatment with acrylic acid at the corresponding concentrations was continued throughout pregnancy and lactation. In each case one male was mated with two females. After 15 days the females were separated from the males and placed on their own. This study revealed a dose-dependent reduction in body weight and in food and water consumption in the F_0 animals of the high and medium dose group, and a decline in the absolute and relative organ weights (heart, liver, kidneys, spleen, brain) in the animals of the F_0 and F_1 generation. In the high dose group of the F_1 generation there was a reduction in body weight-gain, and the fertility index and gestation index were also reduced. In addition, the weights of the foetuses on the 7th and 21st day were lower than for the controls. However, the differences were not significant. At doses of 250 and 83 mg/kg there were no differences from the control animals. Macroscopic and microscopic examinations of the internal organs of all the animals did not show any significant changes in comparison with the corresponding controls (DePass and Weil, 1980, 1983).

7.9 Effects on the immune system
No information available.

7.10 Neurotoxicity
No information available.

7.11 Other effects
Tympany of the stomach and forestomach and the consequent effect (flattening of the mucosal fold of the gastric gland) observed after repeated oral administration of acrylic acid to rats has been interpreted as a consequence of the bacteriocidal action of acrylic acid and its corresponding effects on the gastro-intestinal flora (BASF, 1987a).

Acrylic acid caused a non-protein-sulphhydryl depletion in the stomach after oral administration at concentrations of >0.08% (approx. 4 mg/kg), and to a lesser degree in the forestomach at a concentration of 20% (1000 mg/kg). No such depletion could be detected in the blood and the liver at <8% (400 mg/kg; DeBethizy et al., 1987).

In contrast, Silver and Murphy (1981) found glutathione depletion in the liver after inhalation of acrylic acid.

Miller et al. (1981b) did not find any reaction between acrylic acid and glutathione in vitro (4 mmol acrylic acid to 2 mmol GSH in phosphate buffer for 30 minutes).

Bacteriocidal action was detected in a suspension assay (method according to Heicken) using *Escherichia coli* and *Staphylococcus aureus*. A 0.5 or 1% solution had a bacteriocidal effect after 5–10 minutes (BASF, 1958).

Acrylic acid inhibited the growth of *E. coli* and *Staph. aureus* (minimum inhibiting concentration at pH 6.5, 0.05 mg acrylic acid/ml for *Staph. aureus* and 0.78 mg acrylic acid/ml for *E. coli*). In *E. coli*, acrylic acid disturbed the incorporation of thymidine into DNA and of uracil into RNA (Glombitza and Heyser, 1971).

Acrylic acid is said to be capable of blocking cell proliferation in Pseudomonas (no further details, Verschueren, 1983).

1000 µg acrylic acid/ml nutrient medium reduced the growth of *E. coli* in the logarithmic growth phase by 50%, without affecting cell size (Loveless et al., 1954).

Acrylic acid was also studied in connection with investigations of the liver toxicity of allyl alcohol. In these studies, the livers of anaesthetized male Sprague-Dawley rats were perfused with acrylic acid for 1 hour. As a parameter for liver damage, the oxygen absorption was measured, especially in the periportal region of the liver. There was no difference compared with the controls (Belinski et al., 1986).

In a separate study, rats and mice (age and sex not stated) were exposed to 75 ppm acrylic acid for 6 hours daily, for 5 days, and were treated with radioactive thymidine 18 hours after the last exposure. The aim of the investigation was to determine the effect of acrylic acid on olfactory cell proliferation. This study showed that acrylic acid caused a 17-fold increase of cell proliferation in mice and a 4-fold increase in rats, in comparison with the corresponding controls (no further details; Swenberg et al., 1986).

8.   Experience in humans

A value of 1.04 ppm has been reported as the olfactory threshold level (Hellman and Small, 1974).

In another study, 0.2 mg/m^3 (approx. 0.09 ppm) was reported as the lowest concentration of acrylic acid perceptible by smell;

0.1 mg/m^3 (approx. 0.045 ppm) was no longer perceived (no further details; Grudzinskii, 1988).

Acrylic acid is a strongly corrosive liquid which causes blistering, and has a pungent, penetrating odour. Both in the liquid state and as the vapour or aerosol, it can lead to severe, painful damage of the skin, eyes and mucous membranes, with the consequent effects (Gosselin, 1976; Kühn-Birett, 1980).

No cross-sensitization to acrylic acid was found in six patients who had exhibited hypersensitivity to sealants manufactured on the basis of acrylate and methacrylate (Condè-Salazar et al., 1988).

9.   Threshold limit values

Since 1981, acrylic acid has been included in Section IIb of the German list of MAK values (DFG, 1981).

In the USA, a TLV of 10 ppm or 30 mg/m^3 was published for 1989/90, and it is intended to lower this to 2 ppm, corresponding to 6 mg/m^3 (ACGIH, 1989).

References

ACGIH (American Conference of Governmental Hygienists) Cincinnati, Ohio
Threshold Limit Values and Biological Exposure Indices for 1989/90

Barnes, J.M.
Observations on the effect on rats of compounds related to acrylamide
Brit. J. Ind. Med., 27, 147–149 (1970)

Barrow, C.S.
Toxicology of the nasal passages
Hemisphere, Washington, New York, London, p. 101–122 (1987)

BASF AG, Abteilung Toxikologie
Bericht über die biologische Prüfung der reinen und rohen Acrylsäure
Unpublished report VII/365–366 (1958)

BASF AG, Abteilung Toxikologie
Bericht über die Prüfung der akuten Inhalationsgefahr (akutes Inhalationsrisiko) von Acrylsäure rein an Sprague-Dawley-Ratten
Unpublished report (1979a)

BASF AG, Abteilung Toxikologie
Bericht über die Prüfung der akuten dermalen Toxizität von Acryl-
säure rein an der Rückenhaut weißer Kaninchen
Unpublished report (1979b)

BASF AG, Abteilung Toxikologie
Bestimmung der akuten Inhalationstoxizität LC/50 von Acrylsäure
rein als Dampf
Unpublished report (1980)

BASF AG, Abteilung Toxikologie
Pränatale Inhalationstoxizität von Acrylsäure an Sprague-Dawley
Ratten
Unpublished report (1981)

BASF AG, Abteilung Toxikologie
Prenatal toxicity of acrylic acid after inhalation in Sprague-Dawleys
rats
Unpublished report (1983)

BASF AG, Abteilung Toxikologie
Bericht über die Prüfung der Toxizität von Acrylsäure an Ratten nach
3 monatiger Gabe per Schlundsonde
Unpublished report, Project No. 35C0380/8250 (1987a)

BASF AG, Abteilung Toxikologie
Prüfung der Toxizität von Acrylsäure an Ratten bei 12 monatiger
Gabe über das Trinkwasser
Unpublished report, Project No. 74C0389/8239 (1987b)

BASF AG, Abteilung Toxikologie
Study of a potential carcinogenic effect of acrylic acid in rats after
long-term administration in the drinking water
Unpublished report, Project No. 72C0380/8240 (1989)

Belinsky,S., Badr, M.Z., Kaufman, F.C., Thurman, G.
Mechanism of hepatotoxicity in periportal regions of the liver lobule
due to allyl alcohol – studies on thiols and energy status
J. Pharmacol. Exp. Ther., 238, 1132–1137 (1986)

Boyland, E.
142. Experiments on the chemotherapy of cancer
4. Further experiments with aldehydes and their derivates
Biochem. J., 34, 1196–1201 (1940)

Buckley, L.A., James, R.A., Barrow, C.S.
Differences in nasal cavity toxicity between rats and mice exposed
to acrylic acid vapors
The Toxicologist, 4, 1, Abstract No. 4 (1984)

Carpenter, C.P., Weil, C.S., Smyth, Jr., H.F.
Range-finding toxicity data: List VIII
Toxicol. Appl. Pharmacol., 38, 313–319 (1974)

Clayton, G.D., Clayton, F.E. (eds.)
Patty's Industrial Hygiene and Toxicology
3rd revised ed., Vol. 2C, p. 4954–4955
John Wiley, New York (1982)

Condè-Salazar, L., Guimaraens, D., Romero, L.V.
Occupational allergic contact dermatitis from anaerobic acrylic reac-
tants
Contact Dermatitis, 18, 129–132 (1988)

Cote, I.L., Hochwalt, A., Seidman, I., Budzilovich, G.N., Solomon, I.I.,
Segal, A.
Acrylic acid: Skin Carcinogenesis in ICR/HA Mice – Poster 945
The Toxicologist, 6 (1), 236 (1986)

Curren, R.D.
Test for chemical induction of unscheduled DNA synthesis in primary
cultures of rat hepatocytes (by Autoradiography)
Microbiological Associates, Bethesda, Maryland (1988)
Commissioned by Rohm und Haas Company

DeBethizy, J.D., Udinsky, J.R., Scribner, H.E., Frederik, C.B.
The disposition and metabolism of acrylic acid and ethyl acrylate in
male Sprague-Dawley rats
Fund. Appl. Toxicol., 8, 549–561 (1987)

DePass, L.R., Fowler, E.H., Meckley, D.R., Weil, C.S.
Dermal oncogenicity bioassay of acrylic acid, ethyl acrylate and butyl
acrylate
J. Toxicol. Environ. Health, 14, 115–120 (1984)

DePass, L.R., Weil, C.S.
Acrylic Acid $CH_2=CHCOOH$
Inclusion in the drinking water of rats for one generation of repdro-
duction
Bushy Run Research Center, Pittsburgh, PA 15213
Unpublished Report No. 43–528 (1980)

DePass, L.R., Weil, C.S., Frank, F.R.
Acrylic Acid $CH_2=CH–COOH$
Subchronic toxicity, inclusion in the drinking water of rats for three months
Bushy Run Research Center, Pittsburgh, PA 15213
Unpublished Report No. 43–529 (1980)

DePass, L.R., Woodside, M.D., Garman, R.H., Weil, C.S.
Subchronic and reproductive toxicology studies on acrylic acid in the drinking water of the rat
Drug Chem. Toxicol., 6 (1), 1–20 (1983)

DFG (Deutsche Forschungsgemeinschaft)
Maximale Arbeitsplatzkonzentration 1981
Senatskommission zur Prüfung gesundheitsschädlicher Arbeitsstoffe, Mitteilung XVII
Harald Boldt Verlag, Boppard (1981)

D'Souza W.R., Francis, W.R.
Vehicle and pH effects on the dermal penetration of acrylic acid: in vitro – in vivo correlation
The Toxicologist, 8, 209, Abstract 831 (1988)

EPA (Environmental Protection Agency)
OHM/TADS (1986)

Gage, J.C.
The subacute inhalation toxicity of 109 industrial chemicals
Brit. J. Ind. Med., 27, 1–18 (1970)

Ghanayem, B.J., Maronpot, R.R., Matthews, H.B.
Ethyl acrylate – induced gastric toxicity
II. Structure-toxicity relationship and mechanism
Toxicol. Appl. Pharmacol., 80, 336–344 (1985)

Glombitza, K.W., Heyser, R.
Antimikrobielle Inhaltsstoffe in Algen
4. Mitteilung, Wirkung der Acrylsäure auf Atmung und Makromolekülsynthese bei Staphylococcus aureus und Escherichia coli
Helgoländer wissenschaftliche Meeresuntersuchungen, 22, 442–452 (1971)

Gosselin, R.F., Hodge, H.C., Smith, R.P., Gleason, M.N. (eds.)
Clinical Toxicology of Commercial Products, 4th ed.
Williams and Wilkins, Baltimore (1976)

Grudzinskii, V.Y.
Definition of single maximum allowable concentrations of acrylic and
methacrylic acid in atmospheric air of residential areas
Gig. Sanit., Iss. 9,64–65 (1988)

Hellmann, Th.M., Small, F.
Characterisation of the odor properties of 101 petrochemicals using
sensory methods
J. Air Pollution Control Ass., 24, 979–982 (1974)

IARC (International Agency for Research on Cancer)
Acrylic acid, methyl acrylate, ethyl acrylate and polyacrylic acid
Monographs on the evaluation of the carcinogenic risk of chemicals
to humans 19, 47–71 (1979)

ICI (Imperial Chemical Industries, PLC)
Acrylic acid: in vitro absorption through human and mouse skin
Unpublished Report No. CTL/P/2047 (1988)

Ishidate, Jr., M., Harnois, M.C., Sofuni, R.
A comparative analysis of data on the clastogenicity of 951 chemical
substances tested in mammalian cell cultures
Mutat. Res., 195, 151–213 (1988)

Klimkina, N.V., Breding, Z.N., Sergeev, A.N.
Experimental basis for maximum permissible content of acrylic acid
in reservoir waters
Prom. Zag. Vodolmor, 9, 171–185 (1969)

Kutzman, R.S., Meyer, G.J., Wolf, A.P.
The biodistribution and metabolic fate of ^{11}C-acrylic acid in the rat
after acute inhalation exposure or stomach incubation
J. Toxicol. Environ. Health, 10, 969–979 (1982)

Lijinsky, W., Andrews, A.W.
Mutagenicity of vinyl compounds in Salmonella thyphimurium
Teratogenesis Carcinog. Mutagen., 1, 259–267 (1980)

Little, A.D., Inc.
Evaluation of acrylic acid mouse skin tumor bioassay and DNA
adduct study performed at New York University Medical Center, ADL
Ref: 55846 (1986)

Loveless, L.E., Spoerl, E., Weisman, T.H.
A survey of effects of chemicals on division and growth of yeast and
Escherichia coli
J. Bacteriol., 68, 637–644 (1954)

Majka, J., Knobloch, K., Stetkiewicz, J.
Evaluation of acute and subacute toxicity of acrylic acid
Med. Pr., 25, 427–435 (1974)

McCarthy, K.L., Baarson, K.A., Aardema, M.L., Putman, D.L.
Comparison of in vivo and in vitro cytogenetic assay results on acrylic
acid Rohm and Haas Co
Abstract of the 10th annual meeting of the Environmental Mutagen
Society, 1988, p. 67, Abstr. No. 163 (1988)

Miller, R.R., Ayres, J.A., Jersey, G.C., McKenna, M.I.
Inhalation toxicity of acrylic acid
Fund. Appl. Toxicol., 1, 271–277 (1981a)

Miller, R.R., Ayres, J.A., Rampy, L.W., McKenna, M.I.
Metabolism of acrylate esters in rat tissue homogenates
Fund. Appl. Toxicol., 1, 410–414 (1981b)

Moore, M.M., Amtower, A., Doerr, C.L., Brock, K.H., Dearfield, K.L.
Genotoxicity of acrylic acid, methyl acrylate, ethylacrylate, methyl
methacrylate and ethyl methacrylate in L5178Y Mouse Lymphoma
Cells
Environ. Mol. Mutagen., 11, 49–63 (1988)

Nachreiner, D.J., Dodd, D.E.
Acrylic acid: Acute vapor inhalation toxicity test in rats
Bushy Run Research Center, Project Report 51–577 (1988)

National Research Council
Chemical-Biological Coordination Center (CBCCT)
Summary tables of biological tests, 3, 51 (1951)
Cited in: Clayton and Clayton, Patty's Industrial Hygiene and Toxi-
cology 3rd revised ed., Vol. 2 (1982)

Oesch, F.
Ames-Test an den Substanzen Acrylsäure, Methylacrylat,
Butylacrylat
Pharmakologisches Insitut der Universität Mainz, Juli 1977
Commissioned by BASF AG, Ludwigshafen/Rhein

Parker, D., Türk, J.L.
Contact sensitivity to acrylate compounds in guinea pigs
Contact Dermatitis, 9, 55–60 (1983)

Patty, F.A. (ed.)
Industrial Hygiene and Toxicology
2nd revised ed., Vol. 2, p. 1794
Interscience, New York (1967)

Rao, K.S., Betso, I.E., Olson, K.I.
A collection of guinea pig sensitisation test results – grouped by
chemical class
Drug Chem. Toxicol., 4, 331–351 (1981)

Reynolds, C.H., Frederick, C.B.
Calculations on the reactivity of acrylate anion with biological nuc-
leophiles
The Toxicologist, 8, 52, Abstract 207 (1988)

Sagelsdorf, P., Lutz, W.K., Schlatter, C.
Investigation of the potential for covalent binding of acrylic acid in
vivo after oral and dermal administration, Preliminary results
Report TOXETHZ 1044K, 22. Januar 1988
Commissioned by BASF AG, Ludwigshafen/Rhein

Segal, A., Fedyk, J., Melchionne, S., Seidman, J.
The isolation and characterisation of 2-carboxyethyl adducts following in vitro reaction of acrylic acid with calf thymus DNA and
bioassay of acrylic acid in female Hsd:(ICR)Br Mice
Chem. Biol. Interaction, 61, 189–197 (1987)

Singh, A.R., Lawrence, W.H., Autian, J.
Embryo-fetal toxicity and teratogenic effects of a group of methacry-
late esters in rats
Toxicol., Appl. Pharmacol., 22, 314–315 (1972)
J. Dent. Res., 51, 1632–1638 (1972)

Silver, E.H., Leith, D.E., Murphy, S.D.
Potentiation by triorthotolyl phosphate of acrylate ester – induced
alterations in respiration
Toxicology, 22, 193–203 (1981)

Silver, E.H., Murphy, S.D.
Potentation of acrylate ester toxicity by prior treatment with the carboxylase inhibitor triorthotolyl phosphate (TOTP)
Toxicol. Appl. Pharmacol., 57, 208–219 (1981)

Slott, V.L., Hales, B.F.
Teratogenicity and embryolethality of acrolein and structurally related compounds in rats
Teratology, 32, 65–72 (1985)

Smyth, Jr., H.F., Carpenter, C.P., Weil, C.S., Pozzani, U.C., Striegel, I.A.
Range finding toxicity data: List VI
Am. Ind. Hyg. Assoc. J., 23, 95–107 (1962)

Swenberg, J.A., Gross, E.A., Randall, H.W.
Localization and quantitation of cell proliferation following exposure to nasal irritants
Toxicology of the Nasal Passages (CIIT Conf. Toxicol., 7th Meeting Data 1984, 291–300)
Barrow, Hemisphere (1986)

Tegeris, A.S., Balmer, M.F., Garner, F.M., Thomas, W.C., Murphy, S.R., McLaughlin, J.E., Seymour, J.L.
A 13 week skin irritation study with acrylic acid in 3 strains of mice
The Toxicologist, 8, abstract 504, p. 127 (1988)

Tegeris, A.S., Balmer, M.F., Morton, M.F., Buckley, I.R., Garner, F.M.
13 Week mouse comparative skin irritation study with acrylic acid
Basic Acrylate Monomer Manufacturers, Washington D.C. 20036, 20036–1702
Unpublished report (1987)

Ullmann's Encyclopedia of Industrial Chemistry
5th ed., Vol. A 1, p. 161
VCH, Weinheim (1985)

Union Carbide Corporation (1977)
Toxicology Studies – Acrylic acid, glacial
Ind. Med. and Toxicol. Department
cited in: IARC, 19, 47–71 (1979)

Valencia, R., Brav, D., Kenny, A., Murack, C., Possin, D.,
Thomas, W., Seymour, J.
Drosophila sex-linked recessive lethal assay of acrylic acid
University of Wisconsin, personal communication to Basic Acrylic
Monomer Manufactures Association, Washington, D.C.
Abstract of the 19th annual Meeting of the Environmental Mutagen
Society, 1988, p. 108, Abstr. No. 264 (1988)

Verschueren, K. (ed.)
Handbook of Environmental Data of Organic Chemicals
Van Nostrand Reinhold, New York (1983)

Waegemaekers, T.H., van der Walle, H.D.
α,β-Diacryloxypropionic acid a sensitizing impurity in commercial
acrylic acid
Derm. Beruf und Umwelt, 32, 55–58 (1984)

Weast, R.C. (ed.)
Handbook of Chemistry and Physics
CRC, Boca Raton (1979)

Wiegand, H.J., Schiffmann, D., Henschler, D.
Nongenotoxicity of acrylic acid and n-butyl acrylate in a mammalian
cell system (SHE cells)
Arch. Toxicol., 63, 250–251 (1989)

Windholz, M. (ed.)
The Merck Index, 10th ed.
Merck & Co., Inc., Rahway (1983)

Yang, L.L.
CHO/HGPRT mutation assay
Microbiological Associates, Study No. T 5372.322 (1988)

van de Zande, L., Kunnen, R., Uittewaal, B., van Wijk, R., Bisschop, A.
Effect on hepatic ornithine decarboxylase of some food additives and
synthetic elastomers
Food Addit. Contam., 3, 57–62 (1986)

Zeiger, E., Anderson, B., Haworth, S., Lawlor, T., Mortelmans, K.,
Speck, W.
Salmonella Mutagenicity Tests: III. Results from the testing of 255
chemicals
Environ. Mutagen., 9, Suppl. 9, 1–110 (1987)

o-Phthalodinitrile

1.   Summary and assessment

o-Phthalodinitrile (o-PDN) is to be regarded as poisonous (35–125 mg/kg).

o-PDN is a convulsive poison which, following the absorption of relatively small quantities and after a latent period of hours, may lead to severe epileptic-type convulsions with a duration of minutes. Early symptoms such as giddiness, nausea, vomiting, headache, etc., usually occur. Absorption of o-PDN takes place in practice predominantly via inhalation and/or via uncovered skin, with heavy sweating apparently favouring absorption; oral uptake is also possible.

There are no clear references to cases of chronic poisoning or to permanent injuries following an occurrence of acute poisoning; the degeneration of nerve fibres in the central nervous system described in rats following high doses of o-PDN appears only after a subsequent period of observation lasting several days.

The frequently occurring leukaemias with oral, subcutaneous or cutaneous administration of the product in a long-term study on mice and rats are to be evaluated only with qualification, since the data on control animals and the documentation of the individual results are incomplete.

In the Ames test with *Salmonella typhimurium* as well as in a HGPRT test (V 79 cells) no genotoxic effect is detectable, with or without activation, in any of the strains tested. A micronucleus test is also negative.

Histological investigations have revealed no pathological changes in the brain of a deceased worker after a fatal occurrence of acute poisoning. No clinical-chemical deviations from the norm are found, either, in the case of persons who have experienced an occurrence of o-PDN poisoning, and likewise no adverse EEG changes. Chromsomal examinations of industrially-exposed persons yield no significantly differing results relative to a control group.

In an epidemiological mortality study on workers who have been exposed to o-PDN no increase is found in deaths or malignant diseases.

On the basis of the available data, it is very questionable whether the one case of leucosis observed in the mortality study can be causally linked with o-PDN on the basis of the presumed leucosis-producing effect of o-PDN in the long-term study on rats and mice. Such a link appears rather unlikely, in fact, because the leucosis case observed falls statistically within the expected numerical limits.

A 90-day feeding study in rat including special test programmes to detect neurotoxicity effects is under investigation on behalf of BG Chemie.

2.   Name of substance

2.1 Usual name	o-phthalodinitrile (o-PDN)
2.2 IUPAC-name	1,2-benzodicarbonitrile
2.3 CAS-No.	91-15-6

3.   Synonyms, common and trade names

1,2-dicyanobenzol
o-dicyanobenzene
o-PDN
phthalic acid dinitrile
phthalodinitrile

4.   Structural and molecular formulae

4.1 Structural formula

4.2 Molecular formula $C_8H_4N_2$

5.   Physical and chemical properties

5.1 Molecular mass, g/mol	128.1
5.2 Melting point, °C	141–142 (Thiess, 1968)
5.3 Boiling point, °C	–
5.4 Vapour pressure, hPa	0,04 (at 20 °C) (BASF, 1980)

5.5 Density, g/cm^3	1,24 (at 20 °C) (Weast, 1977/78)
5.6 Solubility in water	sparingly soluble (1 g/litre) (BASF, 1980)
5.7 Solubility in organic solvents	low in ligroin (Weast, 1977/78) and polyethylene glycol (Yoshikawa and Kawai, 1966) good in alcohol, ether, chloroform (Weast, 1977/78) very good in benzene (Weast, 1977/78)
5.8 Solubility in fat	low (BASF, 1980)
5.9 pH-value	no information available
5.10 Conversion factor	1 ppm $\overset{\wedge}{=}$ 4.95 mg/m^3 1 mg/m^3 $\overset{\wedge}{=}$ 0.20 ppm (at 25 °C and 1013 hPa) (Clayton and Clayton, 1978)

6.   Uses

Intermediate product for the manufacture of pigments (BASF, 1980).

7.   Experimental results

7.1   Toxicokinetics and metabolism
No information available.
7.2   Acute and subacute toxicity

Table 1. Acute toxicity

Animal species	Route of exposure (vehicle)	Dose, mg/kg	References
Mouse	ip (aqueous suspension)	LD_{50} approx. 50	Zeller et al., 1969
Mouse	ip (in propylene glycol)	LD_{50} 34.5	Yoshikawa and Kawai, 1966
Mouse	ip (in Tween 20)	LD_{50} approx. 5–10	Nakamura and Ohyanagi, 1965
Mouse	oral	LD_{50} 65.2	Yoshikawa and Kawai, 1966
Mouse	sc (in propylene glycol)	LD_{50} 46.4	Yoshikawa and Kawai, 1966
Mouse	sc (in propylene glycol)	LD_{50} approx. 50	Thiess, 1968
Rat	oral (aqueous suspension)	LD_{50} approx. 125	Zeller et al., 1969
Rat	oral (in propylene glycol)	LD_{50} approx. 35	Thiess, 1968
Rabbit	oral (aqueous suspension)	LD_{50} <25 convulsions	Zeller et al., 1969
Rabbit	oral (in food)	50 : tolerated 100 : convulsions, lethal after 22 hours	Thiess, 1968
Rabbit	oral (in propylene glycol)	12.5: survived 25 : convulsions, 50 : lethal	Thiess, 1968
Rabbit	sc (no data)	10: tolerated 50: convulsions, survived 100: convulsions, lethal after 22 hours	Thiess, 1968

Table 1 (continued)

Animal species	Route of exposure (vehicle)	Dose, mg/kg	References
Rat	cutaneous (aqueous suspension 4 hours/10% to the body surface, abdominal skin)	convulsions	Thiess, 1968
Rabbit	cutaneous (50% aqueous rubbed-on preparation, 20 hours)	up to 5000 tolerated	Zeller at al., 1969; Thiess, 1968
Rat, Mouse	inhalation dynamic	fine dust, just visually detectable, 8 hours, concentrations not determined: convulsions, death after 24 hours	Thiess, 1968
Mouse, Rat, Guinea-pig, Rabbit	inhalation static	sublimation at 170 to 180 °C conc. (calculated) 3–5 mg/litre: mouse death, rat heightened reflexes, guinea-pig sur-vived, rabbit survived	Thiess, 1968
Rat	inhalation	at 20 °C, air enriched with volatile components, 8 hours, no effects	Zeller et al., 1969

Regardless of the different routes of exposure, absorption of o-PDN was followed in all species of experimental animals by balance disturbances, heightend reflexes and convulsions.

According to EEG studies in rabbits, o-PDN apparently inhibits the excitation of the thalamus and midbrain produced by electrical stimulation. Following 60-day application of o-PDN, minor phagoerythematous infiltration and atrophy of the brain cells have apparently been observed histologically (data on the dose and on the type of atrophy observed are lacking; Ito, 1971).

In the brain of rats that received 100 mg/kg ip, no histological changes were observed immediately after dosing; in rats that had been killed 7 days after injection, dosing with 50 and 70 mg/kg produced degenerative changes (silver impregnation) in the nerve fibres of the subthalamus and parts of the mesencephalon (Nakamura and Ohyanagi, 1965).

Cutaneous application of 50 mg/kg 20 times, followed by cutaneous application of 100 mg/kg 21 times, evoked no symptoms of poisoning in cats (Zeller et al., 1969).

7.3   Skin and mucous membrane effects

A 50% aqueous rubbed-on preparation caused no signs of irritation on the shaved dorsal skin of white rabbits after being allowed to exert its effects for 15 minutes and 20 hours, and no irritation was caused, either, to the skin of the ear of rabbits following application of the unmodified product, a 10% aqueous rubbed-on preparation, or a 10% solution in olive oil. (Thien, 1968; Kleinsorge et al., 1979)

No more than slight transient signs of irritation were caused to the mucosa of the eye of rabbits (Thiess, 1968; Kleinsorge et al., 1979).

7.4   Sensitization

No information available.

7.5   Subchronic and chronic toxicity

Oral dosing with 5 mg/kg 25 times (twice a week for 3 months) was tolerated by a cat although it caused vomiting and balance disturbances, whilst dosing once with 20 or 50 mg/kg led to death within a short time (Nakamura and Ohyanagi, 1965).

7.6   Genotoxicity

7.6.1 In vitro

In the Ames test o-PDN was negative with or without metabolic activation in experimental strains TA 100, TA 1535, TA 98 and TA 1537 (BASF, 1978).

o-PDN was dissolved in DMSO (final concentration in the medium 1%) and assessed for its genotoxic potential in the mammalian HGPRT system using Chinese hamster cell line V 79. The cells were exposed to the test substance for four hours at concentrations of 22.3; 90.0; 160.0 and 230.0 µg/ml with and without S9 mix. The highest concentration of the test substance resulted in a cell survival of 86.9% and 90.9% without S9 mix; 92.0% and 80.6% with S9 mix in the two experiments. In two independently performed experiments no genotoxic activity could be detected under the experimental conditions described in the test report mentioned above. The clearly enhanced mutation rates after treatment with the positive control substances ethyl-methane sulfonate (EMS) and 9,10-dimethyl-1,2-benzanthracene (DMBA) demonstrated the sensitivity of the test system (LMP, 1987a).

7.6.2 In vivo

o-PDN was assessed for its genotoxic potential to induce micronuclei in bone marrow cells of the mouse. The doses of the test substance administered per os, twice, separated by 24 hours, were 2; 7; 20 mg/kg b.w. Preparation of bone marrow cells was done 6 hours (high, medium and low dose), 24 hours and 48 hours (high dose only) after the second application of the test substance. Positive control substances (cyclophosphamide and benzene) were administered singly per os. Preparation time was 24 hours after administration of positive control substances. In each experimental group 1,000 cells from each of 10 animals (5 males; 5 females) were scored. In the group treated with benzene 1,000 bone marrow cells of each of 5 males were scored. There was no enhancement of the number of cells with micronuclei in the groups treated with the test substance as compared with the negative controls treated with the solvent. On the other hand, the sensitivity of the test system was demonstrated by significantly enhanced micronuclei rates after treatment with the positive controls (LMP, 1987b).

7.7 Carcinogenicity

To test the carcinogenic activity, 5 male and female mice (CC-57-W strain) and 50 male and female rats (Rapollo breed sterile) received o-PDN orally (in food) 5 times a week, subcutaneously once every 10 days, or dermally in applications over 2 years. In the case of the mice, the o-PDN dose was reduced in the first 5 months because of its toxic effect: for dosing sc, from 2.0 to 1.0, then to 0.5, 0.25 and 0.2 mg/mouse (0.2 mg/mouse sc $\hat{=}$ approx. 1/30 LD_{50}); for dermal application, from 2.0 to 0.8 mg/mouse (0.8 mg/mouse approx. 1/8 LD_{50}) and for oral dosing from 2.0 to 1.0 mg/mouse (1.0 mg/mouse approx. 1/6 LD_{50}). The last mentioned dose in each case was tolerated well and administered for over 1.5 years. Rats received a constant dose of 5 mg/rat, orally and sc, for over 3 years. Calculated per kg body weight, mice (assumed weight 20 g) received approx. 100–50 mg/kg in food, approx. 100–40 mg/kg dermally, and approx. 100–10 mg/kg sc; rats (assumed weight 200 g) approx. 25 mg/kg in food and approx. 25 mg/kg sc. The leukaemias found included perivascular leukaemic infiltrates, poorly differentiated forms of leukaemia and lymphoma-like changes, as well as both lymphatic and myeloid forms of leukaemia, in the lymph nodes, kidneys, liver and spleen of the mice. Similar histological changes also occurred in the rat (see Table 2). There are no data on the frequency of occurrence of tumours in the control groups for mice and rats or on historical controls. It is merely reported that in control mice leukaemias were observed in 6.8% of cases overall (no absolute figures), i.e. 10–12 times fewer than in the experiments. There are no data on the causes of death in the non-experimental mice and rats (Pliss and Volfson, 1972).

7.8   Reproductive toxicity
      No information available.

7.9   Effects on the immune system
      No information available.

7.10 Neurotoxicity
      See 7.2.

7.11 Other effects
      No information available.

8.   Experience in humans

Cases of acute poisoning have been described in o-PDN manufacture following uptake through the skin and following inhalation of the dust; heavy sweating and relatively prolonged skin contact favour percutaneous absorption. The symptoms of poisoning occurred after a mean latency period of about 12 hours (0.5 to 48 hours) and were expressed in the form of giddiness, nausea, retching, vomitting, headaches, loss of consciousness and convulsions. Skin

Table 2. The following tumours were found

| Spe-cies | Route of expo-sure | Experimental animals | | Day of ap-pear-ance of the first tu-mour | Leu-ko-sis | Distribution of the tumours | | | | | | |
		Total	Animals with tumours			Thyroid gland	Mammary gland	Ovaries prostate	In-tes-tine	Li-ver	Mesen-terium	Local
Mouse	food	23	23	457	23					1		
	dermal	27	20	324	19			1				
	subcut.	22	20	443	20							1
Rat	food	18	8	461	6	1	1	1[a]		2	1	
	subcut.	28	22	145	15		3		1	4		1

[a] Prostate

and mucosal irritation were observed (Zeller et al., 1969; Thiess, 1968).

In the case of 81 workers who had been working with o-PDN in the course of their employment (mean exposure period 8.5 years (1 to 34 years)) and among whom 11 had suffered acute o-PDN poisoning, there were no abnormal findings in memory tests, internal and neurological examinations, and in investigations in the clinical-chemistry laboratory (blood status, liver status, urine status); in the case of 15 particularly exposed workers (11 of them having suffered acute poisoning) no adverse EEG results were recorded (Kleinsorge et al., 1979).

The investigations carried out on the brain of one worker following a case of fatal o-PDN poisoning revealed no detectable pathological changes at the histological level (Thiess, 1968).

In an epidemiological mortality study, 83 retired employees who had each been exposed to o-PDN for longer than 6 months were investigated. Against the expected figure of 11.92 for the Federal Republic, the 13 deaths observed in this cohort were still within the statistical limits of variability. The 4 cases of malignant disease observed in total (2 carcinomas of the lung, 1 carcinoma of the stomach, and a myeloid leucosis) did not exceed the expected figures (Frentzel-Beyme et al., 1979).

In the case of 20 industrial workers (ages 32 to 62 years) with a possible o-PDN exposure of 2 to 24 years, chromosomal examinations were carried out on lymphocytes in culture and compared with a corresponding control group. Of the 20 employees examined, 7 had experienced an occurrence of acute o-PDN poisoning. There was no significant observable disparity between the results (Fleig and Thiess, 1979).

9.   Threshold limit values

No information available.

References

BASF AG
Ames-test for o-phthalodinitril
Unpublished investigation (1978)

BASF AG
Data-sheet o-phthalodinitril (1980)

Fleig, J., Thiess, A.M.
Chromosomenuntersuchungen bei Mitarbeitern mit Exposition gegenüber ortho-Phthalodinitril
Zbl. Arbeitsmed., 29, 127–129 (1979)

Frentzel-Beyme, R., Thiess, A.M., Wieland, R.
Mortalitätssurvey bei Mitarbeitern aus der ortho-Phthalodinitril-Produktion
Zbl. Arbeitsmed., 28, 121–127 (1979)

Ito, J.
Experimental study on the neurotoxic action of o-phthalodinitril
Kansai Ika Daigaku Zasshi, 23, 93 (1971,
Cited in: Chemical Abstract, 77, 71015j (1972)

Kleinsorge, H., Thiess, A.M., Zeller, H.
Untersuchungen zur Morbidität bei Mitarbeitern aus der ortho-Phthalodinitril-Produktion
Zbl. Arbeitsmed., 29, 130–132 (1979)

LMP (Laboratory for mutagenicity testing)
o-PDN – Detection of gene mutations in somatic mammalian cells in culture: HGPRT-test with V 79 cells
Technical University Darmstadt, Study 271 A (1987a)

LMP (Laboratory for mutagenicity testing)
o-PDN – Micronucleus test in bone marrow cells of the mouse
Technical University Darmstadt, Study 271 B (1987b)

Nakamura, K., Ohyanagi, H.
Histological studies on the rat brain in case of acute phthalodinitrile intoxication
Kobe J. Med. Sci., 11, 63 (1965)

Pliss, G.B., Volfson, N.I.
Leukosogenic effect of phthalodinitrile
Vop. Onkol., 18, 81–86 (1972)

Thiess, A.M.
Beobachtungen von Gesundheitsschädigungen und Vergiftungen durch Einwirkung von o-Phthalodinitril
Zbl. Arbeitsmed., 18, 303–312 (1968)

Weast, R.C. (ed.)
Handbook of Chemistry and Physics
CRC, Cleveland, Ohio (1977/78)

Yoshikawa, H., Kawai, K.
Toxicity of phthalodinitrile and tetra chlorophthalodinitrile
Ind. Health, 4, 11–15 (1966)

Zeller, H., Hofmann, H.T., Thiess, A.M., Hey, W.
Zur Toxizität der Nitrile
Zbl. Arbeitsmed., 19, 225–238 (1969)

m-Nitroaniline

1. Summary and assessment

On subcutaneous injection in the rabbit, about 15% of the administered m-nitroaniline appears in the urine within 2 days. The excretion of diazo-positive metabolites in the urine is increased on intraperitoneal administration of m-nitroaniline to rats. Up to 77% of m-nitroaniline is absorbed from the small intestine in rats.

The substance is toxic to several animal species (LD_{50} oral, 308–900 mg/kg). Dyspnoea and convulsions are described as symptoms of an acute toxic effect. Autopsies show evidence of asphyxia. m-Nitroaniline causes marked methaemoglobin formation in the rat and the cat.

Repeated subcutaneous administration of sublethal doses (ca. 250 mg/kg, 3 times in 8 days) to rabbits, leads to marked emaciation and severe secondary anaemia. The microscopic changes seen in various tissues are due to haemolysis. Subcutaneous injections of 15 mg/kg to rabbits for 11 days have not caused any overt toxic effects.

m-Nitroaniline is only very slightly irritating to the skin and eyes of rabbits.

m-Nitroaniline has been shown to have mutagenic activity in most of the numerous Salmonella/microsome tests that have been carried out and in the Rec assay on *Bacillus subtilis*, but not in tests with *Escherichia coli*. The UDS test is negative.

m-Nitroaniline does not cause any changes to the liver enzymes in rats after intraperitoneal injection, and therefore probably has no hepatotoxic effects.

It causes no increase in methaemoglobin formation from rat haemoglobin in vitro.

m-Nitroaniline is toxic on acute administration to various species, causing dyspnoea, convulsions and methaemoglobin formation. Repeated subcutaneous injections of sublethal doses to rabbits leads to emaciation and severe secondary anaemia due to haemolysis. m-Nitroaniline is only very slightly irritating to the eyes and skin. The chemical is mutagenic in the *Salmonella*/microsome test and in the Rec assay; further results on genotoxicity are contradictory.

2.   Name of substance ____

2.1	Usual name	m-Nitroaniline
2.2	IUPAC-name	1-Amino-3-nitrobenzene
2.3	CAS-No.	99-09-2

3.   Synonyms, common and trade names _______________________________

m-Nitranilin
m-Nitroaminobenzene
m-Nitrophenylamine
m-Aminonitrobenzene
3-Nitroaniline
3-Nitrobenzenamine
3-Aminonitrobenzene
C.I. 37030

4.   Structural and molecular formulae ________________________________

4.1   Structural formula

4.2   Molecular formula $C_6H_6N_2O_2$

5.   Physical and chemical properties _________________________________

5.1	Molecular mass, g/mol	138.13
5.2	Melting point, °C	114 (Windholz, 1983) 113 (Hoechst, 1988a, b)
5.3	Boiling point, °C	306 (Windholz, 1983)
5.4	Vapour pressure hPa	0.212 (at 100 °C; Ullmann, 1979) 1.333 (at 119 °C; Hoechst, 1983)
5.5	Density, g/cm^3	1.1747 (at 20 °C) (Weast, 1986/87)

5.6 Solubility in water	slight (Windholz, 1983; Hoechst, 1988a, b)
5.7 Solubility in organic solvents	Alcohol, ether, acetone, toluene (Weast, 1986/87; Hoechst, 1988a, b), propylene glycol (Watanabe et al., 1976)
5.8 Solubility in fat	Soluble in olive oil (a 3.5% solution is equivalent to a saturated solution; Wells et al., 1920)
5.9 pH-value	No information available
5.10 Conversion factor	1 ppm $\hat{=}$ 732 mg/m^3 1 mg/m^3 $\hat{=}$ 0.17 ppm (25 °C and 1013 hPa) (at 25 °C and 1013 hPa)

6.   Uses

Intermediate in the manufacture of dyestuffs (Ullmann, 1979).

7.   Experimental results

7.1   Toxicokinetics and metabolism

By means of ether-extraction, m-nitroaniline could be detected and colorimetrically measured in the urine of rabbits in both the conjugated and unconjugated forms following subcutaneous injection. After subcutaneous injection into three rabbits (weight 1.9–2.1 kg) of 530 mg m-nitroaniline (252–279 mg/kg body weight), 61.2, 67.5 and 77.5 mg were found in the urine after 1 day, 5.3, 0 and 21.0 mg after 2 days, and none was detectable after 3 days. About 15% of the injected m-nitroaniline was therefore found in the urine after 2 days by this method (no further information; Wells et al., 1920).

Five male Wistar rats (weight 150–220 g) received a single intraperitoneal injection of 100 μmol m-nitroaniline/kg body weight (dissolved in 2 ml/kg propylene glycol), and their urine and faeces were collected separately for 5 hours. Diazo-positive metabolites were increased 6.8- and 8.2-fold, respectively, compared with the control group (Watanabe et al., 1976).

The small intestines of Sprague-Dawley rats (120–200 g, under anaesthesia) were perfused from the cardiac opening to the end of the ileum with a solution of m-nitroaniline (1 mM/l, equivalent to 138.13 mg/l) together with electrolytes (NaCl, KCl, $CaCl_2$, Na_2HPO_4, NaH_2PO_4). The solution was maintained at 37 °C and the perfusion rate was 1.5 ml/minute. The difference between the amount of substance administered and that at the end of the ileum was analytically determined. In two experiments under these conditions, 77 (±2)% of the chemical was found to be absorbed (Schanker et al., 1958).

7.2   Acute and subacute toxicity

The acute toxicity of m-nitroaniline has been investigated in several species. An overview of the LD_{50} values is given in Table1.

An LD_{50} value of 310 mg/kg was found on oral administration of m-nitroaniline to male CF_1-mice (no further details; Back et al., 1972; Vernot et al., 1977).

After oral administration of m-nitroanliline to male Sprague-Dawley rats, an LD_{50} value of ca. 535 mg/kg was reported (Back et al., 1972; Vernot et al., 1977).

Vasilenko et al. (1974) found an oral LD_{50} value of 900 mg/kg in the rat (no details of strain or sex).

The oral LD_{50} value in guinea-pigs was 450 mg/kg (Sax, 1984).

Table 2 gives an overview of the toxicity of m-nitroaniline to various species on acute administration. In each case, the substance was administered as a 3.5% saturated solution in olive oil (no information given on strain or sex or on number of animals tested). A dog (6.3 kg) died within 4 hours of an intraperitoneal injection of 70mg m-nitroaniline/kg body weight. The lethal intraperitoneal dose for rabbits (weight 1.7–2 kg) was around 430–500 mg/kg, and in most cases, 290–340 mg/kg body weight was lethal after intraperitoneal injection in rabbits (no further information), while 200–250 mg m-nitroaniline/kg body weight was tolerated without visible toxic effects. A cat (weight 2.025 kg) died after intraperitoneal injection of 212 mg m-nitroaniline/kg. In a guinea-pig (weight 0.97 kg), a dose of 206 mg m-nitroaniline/kg was lethal. In all cases, death was preceded by dyspnoea and convulsions, with erythrocyturia, albuminuria and eventually anuria (no haemoglobin or methaemoglobin were found in the urine). At autopsy, macroscopic and microscopic signs of asphyxia were seen. The blood was dark-coloured and clotting time was increased. No methaemoglobin was detected in the blood using spectroscopic methods. The right side of the heart was dilated and the lungs were oedematous (to a greater or lesser extent). There were a few cases of fatty degeneration of the myocardium, focal centro-lobular fatty degeneration in the liver and liver cell necrosis. In the kidneys vacuolation, fatty degeneration and necrosis of the tubule epithelia (particularly in the Henle's loop) were found. In rabbits and dogs haemoglobin in the kidney tubules and protein deposits in the glomeruli were seen due to marked haemolysis (Wells et al., 1920).

Bolt et al. (1985) reported that m-nitroaniline caused marked methaemoglobin formation, and referred to the work of Jung (1947). According to this inadequately-documented work, intraperitoneal injection of 11.4 or 12 mg m-nitroaniline/kg into two cats caused 53 and 50% methaemoglobin formation, respectively, and led to the appearance of Heinz bodies. Maximum toxicity occurred after about 6 hours. Haemolysis was not observed. Both animals survived (Bolt et al., 1985; Jung, 1947).

Oral administration of 450 mg m-nitroaniline/kg body weight to rats caused a significant increase in the level of methaemoglobin in the blood (no further details; Vasilenko et al., 1974).

After a single intraperitoneal injection of 100 μmol m-nitroaniline/kg body weight (dissolved in 2ml/kg propylene glycol) in five male Wistar rats (weight 150–220 g) the methaemoglobin content of the blood was $12.9 \pm 3\%$ after 5 hours (no information given on the methaemoglobin content in the blood of the control animals; Watanabe et al., 1976).

The results presented in Tables 1 and 2 indicate the following descending order of acute toxicity: dog, cat, guinea-pig, rabbit, mouse, rat (Wells et al., 1920; Vasilenko et al., 1974; Back et al., 1972; Vernot et al., 1977; Sax, 1984; Jung, 1947).

After three subcutaneous injections of ca. 250 mg m-nitroaniline/kg (3.5% in oil) within 8 days (total dose 750 mg/kg) a rabbit showed severe emaciation, and haematological tests revealed secondary anaemia. At autopsy, changes in the bone marrow similar to those characteristic of anaemia were diagnosed. The kidneys and spleen were swollen and dark in colour. Microscopic changes resulting from haemolysis were found in the tissues. A rabbit (weight 1.9 kg) tolerated subcutaneous injections of 15 mg m-nitroaniline/kg body weight/day for 11 days (total dose 165 mg/kg body weight) without any overt adverse effects (Wells et al., 1920).

Table 1. Acute toxicity (LD$_{50}$) of m-nitroaniline to various animal species

Species	Strain	Sex	Route of exposure	LD$_{50}$ (mg/kg bw)	References
Mouse	CF$_1$	male	oral	308 (228–416[a])	Back et al., 1972
Mouse	CF$_1$	male	oral	310 (230–420)	Vernot et al., 1977
Rat	Sprague Dawley	male	oral	535 (362–793[a])	Back et al., 1972
Rat	Sprague Dawley	male	oral	540 (360–790[a])	Vernot et al., 1977
Rat	n.s.	n.s.	oral	900	Vasilenko et al., 1974
Guinea-pig	n.s.	n.s.	oral	450	Sax, 1984

n.s. not specified
bw body weight
[a] 95% confidence limits

7.3   Skin and mucous membrane effects

m-Nitroaniline was tested on three rabbits for local irritant effects according to OECD-test guideline no. 404 (1981). Results were recorded at 30 and 60 minutes, and 24, 48 and 72 hours after the end of the 4-hour application period. After 30 minutes, erythema was seen, varying from barely perceptible to marked. This began to clear up after 24 hours and was no longer present after 48 hours (average value for erythema and scab formation 0.1, for oedema formation 0.0). In this study, the skin irritancy of m-nitroaniline was very slight (Hoechst, 1988a).

In another study, the eye irritancy of m-nitroaniline was studied in three rabbits according to OECD test guideline no.405 (1987). Evaluation was carried out 1, 24, 48 and 72 hours after instillation. After 1 hour, the conjunctiva showed clear hyperaemia and slight oedema, which was reversed after 24 hours (average values for reddening, oedema, iritis and clouding of the cornea were 0.0 in all

Table 2. Overview of the acute toxicity of m-nitroaniline to various animal species

Species[a]	Weight	Route of exposure	Dose range tested (mg/kg bw)	Toxic effect[b]	References
Dog	6.3	i.p.	70	lethal within 4 hours	Wells et al., 1920
Rabbit	1.7–2	i.p.	200–250	no visible toxic effects[c]	Wells et al., 1920
Rabbit	1.7–2	i.p.	286–336	mainly lethal[c]	Wells et al., 1920
Rabbit	1.7–2	i.p.	429–504	lethal[c]	Wells et al., 1920
Guinea-pig	0.97	i.p.	206	lethal	Wells et al., 1920
Cat	2.025	i.p.	212	lethal	Wells et al., 1920
Cat	n.s.	i.p.	11.4–12	50–53% methaemoglobin formation	Jung, 1947
Rat	n.s.	oral	450	methaemoglobin formation[c]	Vasilenko et al., 1974

n.s. not specified
bw body weight
[a] Strain and sex of experimental animals not specified
[b] See section 7.2 for further clinical, macroscopic and microscopic findings
[c] Number of animals studied not specified

cases). In this study, the eye irritancy of m-nitroaniline was very slight (Hoechst, 1988b).

Instillation of 10–20 mg m-nitroaniline into the eyes of rabbits did not cause irritation. The presence of 10–20 mg in the eye of an anaesthetized rabbit for 1 hour caused a faint yellow stain and clouding of the cornea (no further details; Grant, 1974).

7.4 Sensitization
No information available.

7.5 Subchronic and chronic toxicity
No information available.

7.6 Genotoxicity

7.6.1 In vitro

m-Nitroaniline (purity >98%) was studied in the Salmonella/microsome test in strains TA 98, TA 100, TA 1535, TA 1537 and TA 1538, with and without a metabolizing system (S9 mix from Aroclor 1254-pretreated rat liver) at eight concentrations ranging from 5 to 1000 µg/plate. The doses used were not toxic to the bacteria. m-Nitroaniline produced dose-dependent reverse mutations in *Salmonella typhimurium* strains TA 98, TA 1535 and TA 1538 with and without metabolic activation, the mutagenic effect being more marked in all cases in the presence of S9 mix (Shahin, 1985).

Shimizu and Yano (1986) also carried out a Salmonella/microsome test with m-nitroaniline (purity ≥ 98%). They used strains TA 98, TA 100, TA 1535 and TA 1538 without metabolic activation. The dose that was toxic to the bacteria was determined, and the mutagenicity test was conducted using a range of doses (0.05–10 mg/plate) of which the highest concentration was bacteriotoxic. m-Nitroaniline was mutagenic to *Salmonella typhimurium* strains TA 98, TA 100, TA 1535 and TA 1538, the effect being dose-related in all cases.

Thompson and co-workers (1983) carried out a Salmonella/microsome test on m-nitroaniline in strains TA 98, TA 100, TA 1535, TA 1537, TA 1538, C 3076, D 3052 and G 46 as well as a mutagenicity test on two tryptophan-deficient strains of *E. coli*, WP2 and WP2uvrA$^-$, with and without metabolic activation (S9 mix from Aroclor 1254-induced rat liver). The highest dose tested was 1000µg/ml agar. Precise details of the concentrations used were not given. Similarly, there was no mention of whether m-nitroaniline was toxic to the bacteria in the dose range tested. m-Nitroaniline was positive in TA 98, TA 100, TA 1535 and TA 1538. The strain most sensitive to the mutagenic effects of m-nitroaniline was TA1538, concentrations of 20–100 µg/ml agar being mutagenic in this strain. The results with *E. coli* were negative (Thompson et al., 1983).

Another Salmonella/microsome test was carried out by Garner and Nutman (1977), using m-nitroaniline at concentrations of 50 and

100 µg/plate in *Salmonella typhimurium* TA 1538 with and without metabolic activation (S9 mix from phenobarbital-pretreated rat liver). m-Nitroaniline was weakly mutagenic in the presence of the metabolizing system (spontaneous mutation rate, 15 revertants/plate; 50µg/plate + S9 mix, 31 revertants/plate; 100 µg/plate + S9 mix, 44 revertants/plate).

Chiu et al., (1978) tested m-nitroaniline at concentrations of 0.1, 1 and 10 µmol/plate in an Ames test in strains TA 98 and TA 100 without the addition of a metabolizing system. At these concentrations, m-nitroaniline had no bacteriotoxic effects and only caused reverse mutations at 10 µmol in strain TA 98.

A further study on the genotoxicity of m-nitroaniline (purity 99.4%) was carried out in the *Salmonella typhimurium* strains TA 98, TA 100, TA 1535, TA 1537 and TA 1538 and in *E. coli* WP2uvrA with and without metabolic activation (S9 mix from Aroclor 1254-induced rat liver). Doses ranging from 4 to 5000 µg/plate were tested. Doses of 5000 and 10,000 µg/plate were toxic to the bacteria. The chemical showed dose-dependent mutagenic activity in strains TA 98, TA 1535 and TA 1538 without metabolic activation. In the presence of a metabolizing system it produced a significant, dose-dependent increase in revertants in strains TA 98, TA 100, TA 1535 and TA 1538 (increase only weak). The results with *E. coli* were also negative in this study (Hoechst, 1983).

m-Nitroaniline was studied in a pre-incubation test at concentrations of 100, 250, 500 and 1000 µg/plate (solvent, DMSO) in *Salmonella typhimurium* strains TA 98 and TA 100 with and without metabolic activation by S9 mix from rat liver. The chemical induced point-mutations in both strains, both with and without metabolic activation. The greatest number of revertants was seen in strain TA98 with the addition of S9 mix (1250 revertants/mg; no further details; Kawai et al., 1987).

In *Salmonella typhimurium* strains TA 98 and TA 100, m-nitroaniline was only mutagenic in the presence of S9 mix from rat liver, while no genotoxic effect was seen without metabolic activation (no further information; Melnikow et al., 1981).

m-Nitroaniline (97% pure) showed no point-mutagenic activity at four concentrations ranging from 0.05 to 0.2 µmol/plate in *Salmonella typhimurium* strains TA 98 and TA 100 in a standard plate test, with and without the addition of S9 mix (containing 10% S9 from Aroclor 1254-induced rat liver). Similarly, m-nitroaniline had no mutagenic effect in a pre-incubation test with the addition of S9 mix containing 20% liver S9 from Aroclor 1254-pretreated hamsters. When flavin mononucleotide (FMN) was added to the pre-incubation medium with hamster S9, facilitating reduction of the nitro group, the chemical was mutagenic at concentrations of 0.1 µmol/plate and above. Similarly, m-nitroaniline was mutagenic from 0.1 µmol/plate in the pre-incubation test with the addition of FMN, if S9 mix from the rat was used for metabolic activation instead of S9 from the hamster. However, the genotoxic activity was less marked with rat S9 than with hamster S9. Mutagenicity in strain TA100 was less evident in each case than in strain TA 98 (Dellarco and Prival, 1989).

Shimizu and Yano (1986) carried out a Rec assay in *Bacillus subtilis* A17 and M45 with various concentrations of m-nitroaniline (detailed information not provided). The highest dose tested (5 µg m-nitroaniline/plate) caused an inhibition zone of 1.5 mm, which was classified as a positive result (more than 1mm was interpreted as positive).

Thompson et al. (1983) performed an autoradiographic study with m-nitroaniline, investigating unscheduled DNA synthesis in hepatocytes prepared by in situ perfusion of the livers of male Fischer rats (weight, 150–170 g). m-Nitroaniline was negative.

7.6.2 In vivo
No information available.

7.7 Carcinogenicity
No information available.

7.8 Reproductive toxicity
No information available.

7.9 Effects on the immune system
No information available.

7.10 Neurotoxicity
No information available.

7.11 Other effects
Five hours after five male Wistar rats (weight 150–220 g) received an intraperitoneal injection of 100 µmol m-nitroaniline/kg body weight (dissolved in 2ml/kg propylene glycol), neither glutamate-oxalate transaminase activity (GOT, 171.6 ± 38.7 Karmen units) nor glutamate-pyruvate transaminase activity (GPT, 35.4 ± 7.5 Karmen units) were significantly different from the control group (GOT, 195.0 ± 22.6, GTP 33.7 ± 6.3 Karmen units). The authors

concluded that m-nitroaniline was not hepatotoxic in the described study (Watanabe et al., 1976).

In an in vitro investigation of methaemoglobin formation, 0.1 µmol haemoglobin from male Wistar rats was incubated for five hours at 37 °C with 0.5µmol m-nitroaniline at pH 6.6. In five separate experiments, methaemoglobin formation (5.1 ± 0.7%) was not significantly different from controls (4.2 ± 1.0%; Watanabe et al., 1976).

8.   Experience in humans

No information available.

9.   Threshold limit values

Maximum concentration in the workplace in Yugoslavia, 0.01 ppm; 0.1 mg/m^3 (Kawai et al., 1987).

References

Back, K.C., Thomas, A.A., MacEwen, J.D.
Reclassification of materials listed as transportation health hazards
Report No. TSA-20-72-3 (1972)
Aerospace Medical Research Laboratory, Ohio

Bolt, H.M., Neumann, H.G., Lewalter, J.
Zur Problematik von BAT-Werten für aromatische Amine
Arbeitsmed. Sozialmed. Präventivmed., 20, 197–201 (1985)

Chiu, C.W., Lee, L.H., Wang, C.Y., Bryan, G.T.
Mutagenicity of some commercially available nitro compounds for
Salmonella typhimurium
Mutat. Res., 58, 11–22 (1978)

Dellarco, V.L., Prival, M.J.
Mutagenicity of nitro compounds in *Salmonella typhimurium* in the presence of Flavin mononucleotide in a preincubation assay
Environ. Mol. Mutagen., 13, 116–127 (1989)

Garner, R.C., Nutman, C.A.
Testing of some azo dyes and their reduction products for mutagenicity using *Salmonella typhimurium* TA 1538
Mutat. Res., 44, 9–19 (1977)

Grant, W.M.
Toxicology of the eye
Charles C. Thomas (ed.), Thomas Books, Springfield, Illinois, USA,
750 (1974)

Hoechst AG, Pharma Forschung Toxikologie und Pathologie
m-Nitroanilin TRTR study of the mutagenic potential in strains of
Salmonella typhimurium (Ames test) and *Escherichia coli*
Unpublished report, No. 83.0011 (1983)

Hoechst AG, Pharma Forschung Toxikologie und Pathologie
m-Nitroanilin TRTR
Prüfung auf Hautreizung am Kaninchen
Unpublished report (1988a)

Hoechst AG, Pharma Forschung Toxikologie und Pathologie
m-Nitroaniline TRTR
Prüfung auf Augenreizung am Kaninchen
Unpublished report (1988b)

Jung, F.
Studien über Methämoglobinbildung
Arch. Exp. Pathol. Pharmakol., 204, 133–156 (1947)

Kawai, A., Gato, S., Matsumato, Y., Matsushita, H.
Mutagenicity of aliphatic and aromatic nitro compounds
Jpn. J. Ind. Health, 29, 34–54 (1987)

Melnikow, J., Keeffe, J.R., Bernstein, R.L.
Carcinogens and mutagens in the undergraduate laboratory
J. Chem. Educ., 58(1), 11–14 (1981)

Sax, N. (ed.)
Dangerous Properties of Industrial Materials
6th ed., p. 2007
Van Nostrand Reinhold, New York (1984)

Schanker, L.S., Tocco, D.J., Brodie, B.B., Hogben, C.A.M.
Absorption of drugs from the rat small intestine
J. Pharmacol. Exp. Ther., 123, 81–88 (1958)

Shahin, M.M.
Mutagenicity evaluation of nitroanilines and nitroaminophenols in
Salmonella typhimurium
Int. J. Cosmet. Sci., 7, 277–289 (1985)

Shimizu, M., Yano, E.
Mutagenicity of mono-nitrobenzene derivatives in the Ames test and rec assay
Mutat. Res., 170, 11–22 (1986)

Thompson, C.Z., Hill, L.E., Epp, J.K., Probst, G.S.
The induction of bacterial mutation and hepatocyte unscheduled DNA synthesis by mono-substituted anilines
Environ. Mutagen., 5, 803–811 (1983)

Ullmanns Encyklopädie der technischen Chemie
4th ed., Vol. 17, p. 398–413
Verlag Chemie, Weinheim (1979)

Vasilenko, N.M., Zvezdai, V.I., Kolodub, F.A.
Toxic action of mono-nitroaniline isomers
Gig. Sanit, 8, 103–104 (1974)
(Chemical Abstract 82:26764 v)

Vernot, E.H., MacEwen, J.D., Haun, C.C., Kinkead, E.R.
Acute toxicity and skin corrosion data for some organic and inorganic compounds and aqueous solutions
Toxicol. Appl. Pharmacol., 42, 417–423 (1977)

Watanabe, T., Ishihara, N., Ikeda, M.
Toxicity of and biological monitoring for 1,3-diamino-2,4,6-trinitro-benzene and other nitro-amino derivatives of benzene and chlorobenzene
Int. Arch. Occup. Environ. Health., 37, 157–168 (1976)

Weast, R.C. (ed.)
CRC Handbook of Chemistry and Physics
57th ed., p. C-96
CRC Press, Boca Raton, Florida (1986/87)

Wells, H.G., Lewis, J.H., Sansum, W.D., MacClure, W.B., Lussky, H.O.
Observations on the toxicity of tetranitromethylaniline (tetryl), tetra-nitroxylene (T.N.X.), tetra-nitraniline (T.N.A.), dinitrodichlorobenzene (parazol) and metanitraniline
J. Ind. Hyg., 2, 247–252 (1920)

Windholz, M. (ed.)
The Merck Index
10th ed., p. 944
Merck, Rahway, USA (1983)

5-Nitro-2-aminotoluene

1. Summary and assessment

There is insufficient data available on 5-nitro-2-aminotoluene for a toxicological evaluation. As far as acute toxicity is concerned, an intraperitoneal LD_{50} of 911 mg/kg has been obtained in male mice.

In the Salmonella/microsome assay with various modifications (with and without S9 mix, addition of Norharman, preincubation) the results are contradictory. The chemical does not induce DNA repair in rat hepatocyte cultures. In the mouse micronucleus test, there are no indications of clastogenic potential.

In man, 5-nitro-2-aminotoluene causes marked methaemoglobin formation.

2. Name of substance

2.1	Usual name	5-Nitro-2-aminotoluene
2.2	IUPAC-name	1-Amino-2-methyl-4-nitroben-zene
2.3	CAS-No.	99-52-5

3. Synonyms, common and trade names

2-Methyl-4-nitroaniline
4-Nitro-o-toluidine
p-Nitro-o-toluidine
2-Methyl-4-nitrobenzenamine
2-Amino-5-nitrotoluene
Ansibases Red RL
Azoene Fast Red GL Base
Azogene Fast Red RL
Daito Red Base RL
Devol Red RL
Diabase Red RL
Fast Red 5NT
Fast Red RL Base

Hiltonil Fast Red RL Base
Kako Red RL Base
Kayaku Red RL Base
Meisei Fast Red RL Base
Mitsui Red RL Base
Naphtoelan Red RL Base
Red Base Ciba X
Red Base Irga X
Red Base NRL
Red RL Base
Spectrolene Red RL
Symulon Red RL Base
Tulabase Fast Red RL
Yamada Fast Red RL Base

4.   Structural and molecular formulae

4.1 Structural formula

4.2 Molecular formula $C_7H_8N_2O_2$

5.   Physical and chemical properties

5.1	Molcecular mass, g/mol	152.16
5.2	Melting point, °C	134–135 at least 127
5.3	Boiling point	No information available
5.4	Vapour pressure	No information available
5.5	Density, g/cm^3	1.1586 (at 20 °C)
5.6	Solubility in water	Very slightly soluble

5.7	Solubility in organic solvents	Soluble in alcohol, ether,
		    acetone, benzene,
		    chloroform

5.8	Solubility in fat	No information available
5.9	pH-value	Approx. 7

5.10 Conversion factor	$1\ ppm \mathrel{\hat=} 6.22\ mg/m^3$

$$1\ ppm \mathrel{\hat=} 6.22\ mg/m^3$$
$$1\ mg/m^3 \mathrel{\hat=} 0.16\ ppm$$
(at 25 °C and 1013 hPa)
(Hoechst; Weast, 1977/78)

6.   Uses

Intermediate product for manufacturing azo dyes and pigments (Hoechst).

7.   Experimental results

7.1   Toxicokinetics and metabolism
No information is available on the toxicokinetics and metabolism of 5-nitro-2-aminotoluene.

In in vitro tests on *Escherichia coli* (strain W 3110), after incubation with 2,5-dinitrotoluene, 5-nitro-2-aminotoluene was demonstrated as the major metabolite by means of thin layer chromatography and mass spectroscopy (Mori et al., 1984).

7.2   Acute and subacute toxicity
The LD_{50} of 5-nitro-2-aminotoluene in the male mouse (NMRI-SPF) after intraperitoneal administration was 911 (563 to 1476) mg/kg (observation period 24 hours). Mice given an intraperitoneal injection of 400 mg/kg showed the following symptoms: loss of balance, paresis and somnolence. These effects began to recede after 3 hours, and after 24 hours the animals were clinically normal (Otto, 1984).

7.3   Skin and mucous membrane effects
No information available.

7.4   Sensitization
No information available.

7.5   Subchronic and chronic toxicity
No information available.

7.6   Genotoxicity
In the Salmonella/microsome assay 5-nitro-2-aminotoluene was tested on strains TA 100, TA 1535, TA 98, TA 1537 and TA 1538, at concentrations of 12.5, 40, 125, 400 and 1250 µg/plate. The metabolising system (S9 mix) was extracted from the livers of male rats which had been pretreated for enzyme induction with

Clophen A 50. At 1500 µg/plate and above, 5-nitro-2-aminotoluene was toxic to the bacteria. In strains TA 1538 and TA 98, 5-nitro-2-aminotoluene showed significant dose-related mutagenic acitivity, both with and without metabolic activation. No clear activating or detoxifying influence of S9 mix could be demonstrated. In strains TA 100, TA 1535 and TA 1537, no mutagenic activity of 5-nitro-2-aminotoluene was evident either with or without S9 mix (Spiegelberg, 1982).

In a further study using a comparable test arrangement (doses not indicated), 5-nitro-2-aminotoluene was mutagenic to strain TA 1535, both with and without S9 mix, and to strain TA 98 with the addition of Norharman (Shimizu and Takemura, 1984).

In contrast, no mutagenic effects were observed in two other studies, also using a comparable test arrangement (Rao, 1987; Kawai et al., 1987).

The substance was tested for the induction of DNA-repair synthesis in isolated rat hepatocytes, at concentrations of 0.01 to 30 mM. In two independent tests there were no indications of an inductive effect (Andrae, 1986).

There was no indication of a clastogenic effect in the micronucleus assay after intraperitoneal administration of 400 mg/kg in mice. This was confirmed by a repetition of the test (Otto, 1982, 1984).

7.7   Carcinogenicity
No information available.

7.8   Reproductive toxicity
No information available.

7.9   Effects on the immune system
No information available.

7.10 Neurotoxicity
No information available.

7.11 Other effects
No information available.

8.   Experience in humans

Pronounced methaemoglobin formation has been observed during the handling of 5-nitro-2-aminotoluene (no further data; Bolt et al., 1985).

9. Threshold limit values

No information available.

References

Andrae, U.
2-Methyl-4-nitroaniline – Test for the induction of DNA repair in rat
hepatocyte primary cultures (study no. HeRe 2-86/BGCH)
Gesellschaft für Strahlen- und Umweltforschung, 1986
Commissioned by BG Chemie

Bolt, H.M., Neumann, H.G., Lewalter, J.
Zur Problematik von BAT-Werten für aromatische Amine
Arbeitsmed. Sozialmed. Präventivmed., 20, 197–201 (1985)

Hoechst AG
Technical Data Sheet

Kawai, A., Goto, S., Matsumoto, Y., Matsushita, H.
Mutagenicity of aliphatic and aromatic nitro compounds
Jpn. J. Ind. Health, 29, 34–54 (1987)

Mori, M.A., Muyahare, T., Hasegawa, Y., Kudo, Y., Kozuka, H.
Metabolism of dinitrotoluene isomers by *Escherichia coli* isolated
from human intestine
Chem. Pharm. Bull., 32, 4070–4075 (1984)

Otto, F.
Testing for mutagenic activity, micronucleus test
Fraunhofer Institut für Toxikologie und Aerosolforschung (1982,
1984)
Commissioned by BG Chemie

Rao, T.K. (1984, personal communication)
Cited in: Walsh, D.B., Claxton, L.D.
Computer-assisted structure-activity relationship of nitrogenous cy-
clic compounds tested in Salmonella assays for mutagenicity
Mutat. Res., 182, 55–64 (1987)

Shimizu, H., Takemura, N.
Mutagenicity of some aniline derivatives
Occup. Health Chem. Ind. Proc. Int. Congr., 11th, 497–506 (1984)

Spiegelberg, T.
Kurzzeitteste auf mutagene Wirksamkeit: Salmonella/Mikrosomen-
Test (nach Ames) mit 5-Nitro-2-Aminotoluol
Fraunhofer Institut für Toxikologie und Aerosolforschung (1982)
Commissioned by BG Chemie

Weast, R.C. (ed.)
Handbook of Chemistry and Physics, C-549
CRC-Press, Cleveland, Ohio, 1977/78

p-Nitrosophenol

1. Summary and assessment

p-Nitrosophenol is quickly absorbed after oral administration to rats (maximum blood level after 1 hour). At higher doses binding to serum proteins is likely to occur. Excretion occurs via the urine (62% after 24 hours, ca. 81% after 7 days) and the faeces (ca. 15% after 7 days). Total excretion after 7 days is ca. 97%. 6% of the dose is excreted in the bile. At least five metabolites are present in the urine, the major one being the glucuronide of 4-aminophenol. p-Nitrosophenol is also absorbed dermally (17.6%). Following dermal application, excretion again occurs in the urine and faeces (ca. 17.4% and 1.1%, respectively, after 7 days).

p-Nitrosophenol is of low acute toxicity on oral administration (LD_{50} rat 300 to 500 mg/kg), whilst no acute inhalation risk from the vapour has been identified. In comparison with aniline, the chemical does not have a particularly strong effect on methaemoglobin-formation in cats. On the other hand, methaemoglobin is observed in rats after repeated oral administration of 32 mg/kg. Repeated oral doses of between 45 and 180 mg/kg given to rats for 28 days produce damage to the mucous membranes of the mouth as well as isolated damage to the kidneys. The NOEL is 5 mg/kg body weight.

Early studies reported that p-nitrosophenol caused slight skin irritation and severe eye irritation, but this is not seen in later investigations that comply with modern test requirements. No data are available on sensitization.

In a subchronic study in rats given 1 mg/kg body weight orally, no methaemoglobin-formation was observed, but activity at this dose level is not to be expected. Other parameters were apparently not investigated.

Variable results have been obtained in mutagenicity tests with p-nitrosophenol. In the Salmonella/microsome test the chemical shows predominantly weak mutagenic activity. It is inactive in Saccharomyces cerevisiae, and similarly in the DNA-repair test and in the DNA-binding test the chemical gives negative results. A cell transformation assay is also negative. In contrast, p-nitrosophenol is clastogenic to rat liver chromosomes in vitro and in the micronucleustest in vivo.

Data on other effects are scanty and restricted to the influence of p-Nitrosophenol on the nitrosation of amines.

In man, transient skin irritation and discolouration of the skin is observed in association with p-nitrosophenol.

2.   Name of substance

2.1 Usual name   p-Nitrosophenol
2.2 IUPAC-name   4-Nitrosophenol
2.3 CAS-No.   104-91-6

3.   Synonyms, common and trade names

1-Hydroxy-4-nitrosobenzene
p-Benzoquinone monooxime
1,4-Benzoquinone oxime
p-Quinone monooxime
Quinone oxime

4.   Structural and molecular formulae

4.1 Structural formula

4.2 Molecular formula $C_6H_5O_2N$

5.   Physical and chemical properties

5.1 Molecular mass, g/mol   123.1
5.2 Melting point, °C   110 (decomposition;
                                     Hoechst, 1978)
                                   144 (for the pure substance
                                   after recrystallization; Weast,
                                   1981/82)

5.3 Boiling point, °C   –

5.4 Vapour pressure	–
5.5 Density, g/cm^3	ca. 0.5 (at 20 °C; Hoechst, 1978)
5.6 Solubility in water	ca. 9 g/l (at 20 °C; Hoechst, 1985)
5.7 Solubility in organic solvents	Alcohol, ether, acetone, benzene (Weast, 1981/82)
5.8 Solubility in fat	No information available
5.9 pH-value	ca. 3 (100 g/l suspension in water; Hoechst, 1985)
5.10 Conversion factor	1 ppm $\hat{=}$ 5.11 mg/m^3 1 mg/m^3 $\hat{=}$ 0.2 ppm (at 25 °C and 1013 hPa)

6. Uses

Intermediate in dyestuff production, vulcanization accelerator, stabilizer in distillation of styrene (Neumüller, 1977).

7. Experimental results

7.1 Toxicokinetics and metabolism

^{14}C-p-Nitrosophenol was administered orally to groups of six Wistar rats (SPF, 200 ± 20 g) as a 0.4% aqueous preparation in carboxymethyl cellulose in single doses of either 100 mg (group I) or 10mg (group II). In group I, a maximum blood level of 60.8 ppm was attained after 25 minutes, while in group II a maximum level of 6.93 ppm was reached after 15 minutes. During the first hour the profiles were similar, and varied like the dose by a factor of about ten. Later, however, the levels after the high dose were proportionally higher, suggesting transient binding to serum proteins at the later sample times. The blood levels calculated related to radioactivity in groups I and II, respectively, were 10.82 ppm and 0.59 ppm after 24 hours, 10.03 ppm and 0.55 ppm after 48 hours, 8.98 ppm and 0.5 ppm after 72 hours and 6.45 ppm and 0.39 ppm after 7 days. The highest activities were found in the liver, kidneys, spleen and lungs by autoradiography 8 hours after administration of the higher dose. After 24 hours the distribution was similar, but the intensity was reduced. After 7 days, slight residual levels were found in the adrenal glands (0.54 ppm), spleen (1.15 ppm), kidneys (1.94 ppm), liver (1.97 ppm) and blood (7.85 ppm). The relatively high blood content was thought to be due to binding to serum proteins. p-Nitrosophenol is mainly eliminated in the urine. Around 62% of the administered dose (100 mg/kg) was eliminated after 24 hours, and 80.85% after 7 days. By the 7th day after administration, 14.91% had been excreted in the faeces, most of this within the first 48 hours. Elimination through the lungs was only 0.26%. The total amount of radioactivity accounted for after 7 days was 96.59%. About 6% was eliminated in the bile. At least five compounds other than p-nitrosophenol could be identified in the urine by thin layer chromatography. The main metabolite detected (ca. 60%) was the glucuronide of 4-aminophenol. In vitro studies showed that p-nitrosophenol can also react with compounds which contain sulphhydryl groups, such as glutathione, cysteinyl glycine, cysteine and N-acetylcysteine. The chromatographic properties of these compounds were similar to the polar metabolites, which could not be identified (NATEC, 1987).

Only about 17.6% of a single dose (100 mg/kg) of p-nitrosophenol applied dermally to rats for 8 hours was absorbed. The blood content 1 to 10 hours after application formed a wide plateau, with a maximum of 0.46 ppm. After 7 days, 17.42% of the applied dose had been eliminated in the urine and 1.08% in the faeces (NATEC, 1989).

7.2   Acute and subacute toxicity

The acute oral toxicity of p-nitrosophenol in male and female Sprague-Dawley rats (number not specified) was assessed over a 7-day observation period. Aqueous suspensions of 0.5 to 16% were administered. The LD_{50} value was ca. 0.5 g/kg. Symptoms of toxicity included spasms, and methaemoglobin was positive (no further details). At autopsy, irritation of the gut was observed (BASF, 1964).

In another study on 30 male white rats (no further details) an oral LD_{50} value of 320 mg/kg was determined. The methaemoglobin content of the blood was measured before treatment, and at 1, 3, and 24 hours and 2, 3, 5, 10, 15 and 20 days after treatment in the surviving animals. A maximum methaemoglobin level of 46.25% was reached 3 hours after administration, and anaemia developed at the same time which persisted for 2 days (no further details). The methaemoglobin levels were 35.18% after 24 hours, 13.28% after 2 days, 11.28% after 3 days, 6.58% after 5 days, 2.86% after 10 days, 1.02% after 15 days and 1.63% after 20 days (Zaitseva, 1973).

A further oral LD$_{50}$ value of 456 mg/kg for male Wistar rats has been reported (Hoechst, 1985).

The acute dermal toxicity of p-nitrosophenol was studied in accordance with OECD test guidelines No. 402 (1981). A dose of 2000mg/kg was applied to groups of five male and five female Sprague-Dawley rats (200–240 g). All the animals survived the 14-day observation period without symptoms or local effects (Safepharm, 1989a).

In an inhalation-risk test at 20 °C, 11 Sprague-Dawley rats which had been exposed once for 8 hours showed no symptoms at the end of the 8-day observation period. Methaemoglobin was negative immediately after exposure. No notable findings were made on autopsy (BASF, 1964).

Two female cats (ca. 3.7 kg) were given a single oral dose by stomach tube of 50mg p-nitrosophenol/kg (purity 87.1%) in sesame oil. The blood methaemoglobin content was determined after 10 and 30 minutes, and after 1, 6 and 24 hours. A weak cyanosis was observed 30 minutes after exposure, and this had clearly worsened after a further 30 minutes. Panting, decreased spontaneous activity and lying on the stomach or side were also observed. Both cats vomited, one after an hour, the second after 4 hours. One cat died after one day. After 30 minutes the methaemoglobin concentrations were 27 and 14%, and after 6 hours methaemoglobin was no longer detectable. Heinz bodies were also increased to a maximum of 13% or 24% after 6 hours. In the surviving cat, the number of reticulocytes reached a maximum of 108 per 1000 after 3 days, and had returned to normal by day 7. A post-mortem on the dead cat revealed pale-coloured kidneys, slight marks on the liver lobes and dark red gastric mucosa with petechial bleeding (Hoechst, 1986).

Male white rats (no further details) were given 1/10 of the LD$_{50}$ (equivalent to 32 mg/kg) 20 times by stomach tube. The treatment caused methaemoglobinaemia, which reached a maximum (25%) after 7 days. The level then stabilized at arount 20% where it remained until the end of the study. Five days after the end of the study, the methaemoglobin level was within the normal range (Zait-seva, 1973).

A 4-week study was carried out to investigate the subacute oral toxicity of p-nitrosophenol (OECD method No. 407, 1981). Five male and five female SPF-Wistar rats received 5 or 15 mg/kg seven times a week by stomach tube. A further group of ten male and ten female rats received 45 mg/kg, which was increased to 90 mg/kg after 15 days and 180 mg/kg after 22 days. No mortality or symptoms of toxicity occurred. Body-weight gain, food intake and ophthalmoscopic findings were similar to controls. In the course of the study, there was a slight reduction in the number of erythrocytes and the haemoglobin level in the male rats and a slight decrease in the partial thromboplastin time in the 45, 90, 180 mg/kg group. The latter effect was also seen in the females. At the same dose, a slight fall in blood urea was seen in the males, and there was a slight decrease in total serum proteins and a slight increase in serum chloride in both sexes. These effects were regarded as treatment-related. In addition, the urine of the females in the 45, 90, 180 mg/kg group contained increased transitional epithelia. At autopsy, the absolute and relative thymus weights in male rats of the 45, 90, 180 mg/kg group were significantly reduced. Macroscopic and microscopic examination revealed gastritis and stomach ulcers in all rats of the 45, 90, 180 mg/kg group and slight chronic gastritis in a female in the 15 mg/kg group. In addition, there were degenerative and regenerative changes in the kidney tubules in three animals of the 45, 90, 180 mg/kg group. The no-effect-level was 5 mg/kg (RCC, 1987).

7.3   Skin and mucous membrane effects

A 50% aqueous preparation of p-nitrosophenol was applied on a patch to the dorsal skin of two white Viennese rabbits. The exposure times were 1, 5 and 15 minutes and 20 hours. No signs of irritation were observed after exposures of 1 to 15 minutes. After a 20-hour semi-occlusive application, slight reddening of the skin and yellow-brown staining of the application site were seen 24 hours and 8 days later (BASF, 1964).

On instillation of 50 µl (poured volume) of the undiluted product into the conjunctival sac of rabbits' eyes, assessment after 1 and 24 hours revealed inflammation and slight reddening of the conjunctiva, slight (1hr) to severe (24hr) clouding of the cornea and very marked oedema. In addition, bleeding of the conjunctiva was seen after 24 hours. After 8 days the findings were unaltered, except that a purulent secondary infection had set in (BASF, 1964).

7.4   Sensitization

The skin sensitizing potential of p-nitrosophenol was tested on female white Dunkin-Hartley guinea-pigs (346–427 g) in a maximization test, in accordance with OECD guideline No.406 (1981). The following solutions or suspensions in distilled water were used: intradermal induction, 0.1% (w/v); local induction, 50% (w/w); local challenge, 50% (w/w). No skin sensitization was observed in any of the 20 animals (Safepharm, 1989 b).

7.5   Subchronic and chronic toxicity

Male white rats were given 1 mg p-nitrosophenol/kg by stomach tube daily for 6 months (no further details). Methaemoglobin levels were similar to those of the controls. Further information was not provided (Zaitseva, 1973).

7.6   Genotoxicity

7.6.1 In vitro

An Ames test was carried out on p-nitrosophenol in strains TA 1530, TA 1535 and TA 1538 without metabolic activation. No mutagenic activity was seen in strains TA 1530 or TA 1535 in the dose range 10–100 µg/plate. In contrast, a 1.8-fold increase in revertants was seen in strain TA 1538 at 30 µg/plate and a 2.6-fold increase at 50 µg/plate. These concentrations were however cytotoxic (Gilbert et al., 1980).

In a further study, p-nitrosophenol (purity 97–98%) was used in a Salmonella/microsome test in strains TA 1535, TA 1537, TA 1538, TA 98 and TA 100 at a range of doses from 20 to 5000 µg/plate. The study was carried out with and without metabolic activation (S9 mix from Aroclor 1254-induced rat liver). Without metabolic activation, weak mutagenic activity was observed only in TA 98 at 100 µg/plate. With metabolic activation, a weakly positive dose-dependent effect took place in strains TA 98 and TA 1537. At 750 µg/plate the number of revertants was increased maximally by a factor of 2.7 in TA 98 and by a factor of 4 in TA 1537. No increase was seen in the remaining strains. Bacteriotoxic effects occurred above 100 µg/plate without S9 mix, and between 500 and 2500 µg/plate with S9 mix (BASF, 1981).

A third Salmonella/microsome test was carried out on strains TA 98 and TA 100 with and without metabolic activation. The p-nitrosophenol used was more than 98% pure. A dose range of from 12.5 to 800 µg/plate was tested. In strain TA 98 without metabolic activation, the number of revertants was increased by at least 2.5-fold over the control level from a dose as low as 25 µg/plate, while in TA 100 this occurred first at 200 µg/plate. Concentrations of 400 µg/plate and above (without metabolic activation) and 800 µg/plate and above (with metabolic activation) were cytotoxic (Shell, 1980; Dean et al., 1985).

Finally, p-nitrosophenol (purity 60%) was studied in the Salmonella/microsome test both with and without metabolic activation (S9 mix from rat and hamster liver cells) in strains TA 100, TA 1535, TA 97 and TA 98. The concentrations used were between 0 and 666 µg/plate. In strain TA 100, p-nitrosophenol was weakly mutagenic without metabolic activation at 333 µg/plate (factor 1.6) and with metabolic activation at 666 µg/plate (factor 1.8). In strains TA 1535 and TA 97 no mutagenic activity was detected with or without metabolic activation, at up to 666 µg/plate. In strain TA 98, there was weak activity (247 µg/plate, factor 2) without metabolic activation and a somewhat stronger effect (666 µg/plate, factor 2.7) with metabolic activation (Zeiger et al., 1988).

p-Nitrosophenol is not mutagenic in *Sacchararomyces cerevisiae* JD1 at concentrations of up to 5 mg/ml, with or without metabolic activation (S9 mix; Shell, 1980; Dean et al., 1985).

When rat liver cells (RL_4-cell cultures) were incubated with p-nitrosophenol at concentrations of 0.75, 1.5 and 3µg/ml, there was an increase in chromatid gaps and a dose-dependent increase in sister chromatid exchange and chromosomal breaks after 24 hours (Shell, 1980; Dean et al., 1985).

In a special Rec-assay with a rec^- mutant from *Bacillus subtilis* and a corresponding rec^+ wild form, p-nitrosophenol (50 µl of a 10^{-2} M aqueous solution, pH1) caused DNA damage (Natake et al., 1979).

p-Nitrosophenol has also been tested for its influence on DNA-repair/synthesis in primary rat hepatocyte cultures. The study was carried out at doses of from 10 µM to 30 mM, with three independent experiments. p-Nitrosophenol showed no genotoxic activity in this system (GSF, 1986).

7.6.2 In vivo

In a micronucleus test, male and female NMRI mice (2.5 to 4 months old) received a single dose, by stomach tube, of 250 mg p-nitrosophenol/kg as a suspension in methocel. In preliminary experiments this dose caused no deaths but produced clear toxic effects within the first 6 hours. The animals were killed after 24, 48 and 72 hours, and 1000 polychromatic erythrocytes per mouse were screened for micronuclei. In addition, the number of micronuclei in 1000 normochromatic erythrocytes was determined. The number of cells containing micronuclei was increased after 24 and 48 hours. The highest value (two evaluations, 0.82 and 0.91%) was recorded after 24 hours, after 48 hours it was 0.38%, and after 72 hours the figure was in the range of control values (0.24%). In addition, the proportion of polychromatic to normochromatic erythrocytes was atypical (1000 PE/1397 NE; control 1000 PE/905 NE after 48 hours). A toxic effect on the spindle could be discounted because only 7% of the evaluated micronuclei were a quarter or more of the diameter of the erythrocyte cytoplasm. Based on these studies, p-nitrosophenol has been classified as clastogenic (LMP, 1983/1988).

A DNA-binding study has also been carried out. Groups of four Wistar rats were given single doses by stomach tube of 15 or 150 mg ^{14}C-labelled p-nitrosophenol/kg. After 6 and 24 hours, DNA and associated proteins were isolated from the liver and stomach of two rats, and were then purified for measurement of the radioactivity. That of the low dose was only just detectable. At the high dose, 80% of the radioactivity was eluted from the stomach with the normally occurring nucleotides (this was therefore natural incorporation and not alkylation). The remaining 20% of labelled DNA could in principle have been nucleotide-nitrosophenol adducts, but DNA activity in the in vitro control showed a similar order of magnitude. The covalent binding index (CBI) for liver and stomach was < 0.2 and was therefore about 50,000 times lower than that of aflatoxin B_1 and 7500 times lower than that of N-methyl-N'-nitro-N-nitrosoguanidine. On this basis, p-nitrosophenol showed no DNA-binding activity in this *in vivo* study (Institute of Toxicology, 1987).

7.7   Carcinogenicity

p-Nitrosophenol (>98% pure, dissolved in methanol) was also studied in a cell transformation test in vitro, using C3H10T1/2-mouse fibroblasts with and without a promoter system (12-O-tetradecanoyl-phorbol-13-acetate). Evaluation took place 3–4 weeks after the treatment. A concentration of 1 µg/ml inhibited cell growth by about 50%, and was used as the highest dose. Other test concentrations were 0.5 and 0.25 µg/ml. p-Nitrosophenol showed no cell-transforming activity either with or without promoter at the dose levels tested (Shell, 1983).

7.8   Reproductive toxicity
No information available.

7.9   Effects on the immune system
No information available.

7.10 Neurotoxicity
No information available.

7.11 Other effects

In an in vitro study it was shown that in the nitrosation of diethylamine p-nitrosophenol can promote the formation of nitrosamines over a wide pH range (2 to 6, maximum at 3 to 5; Walker et al., 1979).

Other work has shown that p-nitrosophenol increases the nitrosation of proline in vivo (rats) and in vitro by factors of 12.2 and 18.2 respectively (Pignatelli, 1982).

8.   Experience in humans

Discolouration of the skin has been reported after contact with p-nitrosophenol. Transient skin irritation was observed at one time due to dust-formation during handling, but this has not occurred since technical protective measures have been in operation (BASF, 1982, 1989). No further information is available.

9.   Threshold limit values

No information available.

References

BASF AG
Gewerbetoxikologische Vorprüfung von p-nitrosophenol
Unpublished report of 29. 12. 1964

BASF AG, Toxicology department
Bericht über die Prüfung von p-nitrosophenol im Ames-Test
Unpublished report of 25. 8. 1981

BASF AG
Written communication of 23. 7. 1982

BASF AG, Company Medical Service
Letter of 1. 9. 1989

Dean, B.J., Brooks, T.M., Hodson-Walker, G., Hutson, D.H.
Genetic toxicology testing of 41 industrial chemicals
Mutat. Res., 153, 57–77 (1985)

Gilbert, P., Rondelet, J., Poncelet, F., Mercier, N.
Mutagenicity of p-nitrosophenol
Fd. Cosmet. Toxicol., 18, 523–525 (1980)

GSF (Gesellschaft für Strahlen- und Umweltforschung, D-8042 Neu-
herberg/München, Institut für Toxikologie)
p-Nitrosophenol – Test for the induction of DNA repair in rat hepatocyte primary cultures
Unpublished report of 5. 2. 1986
Commissioned by BG Chemie

Hoechst AG
Technical data sheet (1978)

Hoechst AG
Safety data sheet p-nitrosophenol (1985)

Hoechst AG, Pharma Forschung Toxikologie und Pathologie
p-Nitrosophenol TF, Wirkung auf das Blutbild (Methämoglobin- und
Heinzkörperbildung) an weiblichen Katzen
Unpublished report of 8. 10. 1986
Comissioned by BG Chemie

Institute of Toxicology, Swiss Federal Institute of Technology and
University of Zürich, CH-8603 Schwerzenbach, Switzerland
Investigation of the potential for covalent binding by p-nitrosophenol
to DNA of rat liver and stomach
Unpublished report of 2. 10. 1987
Commissioned by BG Chemie

LMP (Laboratorium für Mutagenitätsprüfung an der Technischen
Hochschule Darmstadt)
Mikrokerntest mit p-nitrosophenol
Unpublished report of 10. 5. 1983 with supplement of 22.4. 1988
Commissioned by BG Chemie

Natake, M., Danno, G., Maeda, T., Kawamura, K., Kanazawa, K.
Formation of DNA-damaging and mutagenic activity in the reaction
systems containing nitrite and butylated hydroxyanisole, tryptophan,
or cysteine
J. Nutr. Sci. Vitaminol., 25, 317–322 (1979)

NATEC-Institut für Naturwissenschaftlich-technische Dienste
GmbH, D-2000 Hamburg 50
Biokinetics and metabolic fate of 4-nitrosophenol in young adult
male rats
Commissioned by BG Chemie (1987/89)

Neumüller, O.-A. (ed.)
Römpps Chemie Lexikon
7th edition, p. 1536 (1977)
Franckh'sche Verlagshandlung, Stuttgart

Pignatelli, B., Bereziat, J.-C., Descotes, G., Bartsch, H.
Catalysis of nitrosation in vitro and in vivo in rats by catechin and
resorcinol and inhibition by chlorogenic acid
Carcinogenesis, 3, 1045–1049 (1982)

RCC (Research and Consulting Company AG)
Subacute 28-day oral toxicity (gavage) study with p-nitrosophenol
TF in the rat
Unpublished report Project No. 047856 commissioned by BG
Chemie (1987)

Safepharm Laboratories Limited, P.O. Box No. 45, Derby, DE1 2BT,
U.K.
Acute dermal toxicity (Limit Test) in the rat
Unpublished report (1989 a)

Safepharm Laboratories Limited, P.O. Box No. 45, Derby, DE1 2BT,
U.K.
Magnusson-Kligman Maximisation study in the guinea pig
Unpublished report (1989 b)

Shell Research Ltd., London
Toxicity studies with base chemicals: *in vitro* genotoxicity studies with
p-nitrosophenol
Unpublished report (1980)

Shell Research Ltd., London
Toxicity studies with base chemicals: in vitro transformation studies
with p-nitrosophenol
Unpublished report (1983)

Walker, E.A., Pignatelli, B., Castegnaro, M.
Catalytic effect of p-nitrosophenol on the nitrosation of diethylamine
J. Agric. Food Chem., 27, 393–396 (1979)

Weast, M. (ed.)
Handbook of Chemistry and Physics, C 437
CRC, Boca Raton, Florida (1981/82)

Zaitseva, N.V.
Besonderheiten der toxischen Wirkung von Nitrosophenol in einem
sanitär-toxikologischen Experiment (German translation)
Nauchn. Trudy, Permskii Politek. Inst., 141, 114 (1973)

Zeiger, E., Anderson, B., Haworth, S., Lawlor, P., Mortelmans, K.
Salmonella mutagenicity tests IV. Results from the testing of 300
chemicals
Environ. Mol. Mutagen., 11, Suppl. 12, 1–158 (1988)

Propargyl alcohol

1. Summary and assessment

On the basis of the existing studies, propargyl alcohol is acutely toxic to animals following oral, dermal and inhalation exposure (LD_{50} rats oral, 20 to 110 mg/kg; LD_{50} rabbits dermal, 16 to 88 mg/kg; LC_{50} rats, 1 hour exposure, about 2.6 mg/l).

An enriched atmosphere at 20 °C leads to the deaths of exposed rats within a few minutes.

Propargyl alcohol has an irritant to corrosive effect on the skin and eyes of animals, an effect which increases with increasing concentration.

Sub-chronic oral and inhalation exposure of animals to propargyl alcohol leads to liver and kidney damage. Bleeding occurs in several organs, irrespective of the route of administration.

In Salmonella/microsome tests, propargyl alcohol shows no evidence of mutagenic activity in strains TA 98, TA 100, TA 1535, TA 1537 and TA 1538.

The German TLV has been 2 ppm ($\hat{=}$ 5 mg/m^3) since 1969.

Experiments are presently being conducted for the Employment Accident Insurance Fund of the Chemical Industry (BG-Chemie) on subchronic inhalation toxicity and mutagenicity.

2. Name of substance

2.1 Usual name	Propargyl alcohol
2.2 IUPAC-name	2-Propyne-1-ol
2.3 CAS-No.	107-19-7

3. Synonyms, common and trade names

Acetylene carbinol
Ethenyl methanol
Ethynyl carbinol
Propyne-(1)-ol-(3)
Propyne-(2)-ol
2-Propynol-1
1-Propyne-3-ol

4.   Structural and molecular formulae

4.1   Structural formula $HC{\equiv}C{-}CH_2OH$

4.2   Molecular formula C_3H_4O

5.   Physical and chemical properties

5.1	Molcecular mass, g/mol	56.06
5.2	Melting point, °C	−48 to −52 (Clayton and Clayton, 1982)
5.3	Boiling point, °C	114–115 (Clayton and Clayton, 1982)
5.4	Vapour pressure, hPa	15.5 (at 20 °C) (Clayton and Clayton, 1982) 28 (at 30 °C) (Hommel, 1985)
5.5	Density, g/cm^3	0.9715 (at 20 °C) (Clayton and Clayton, 1982)
5.6	Solubility in water	Fully miscible (Clayton and Clayton, 1982)
5.7	Solubility in organic solvents	Soluble in benzene, chloroform, 1,2-dichloroethane, ethanol, ether, acetone, dioxane, tetrahydrofuran, pyridine; insoluble in aliphatic hydrocarbons (Clayton and Clayton, 1982)
5.8	Solubility in fat	No information available
5.9	pH-value	No information available
5.10	Conversion factor	1 ppm $\overset{\wedge}{=}$ 2.29 mg/m^3 1 mg/m^3 $\overset{\wedge}{=}$ 0.44 ppm (at 25 °C and 1013 hPa)
5.11	Odour	Mild and geranium-like (Bayer, 1984)

6. Uses

Corrosion inhibitor, solvent for cellulose acetate, polishing agent in galvanotechnics, stabilizer for chlorinated hydrocarbon formulations, herbicide, intermediate in organic syntheses (Falbe et al., 1985).

7. Experimental results

7.1 Toxicokinetics and metabolism

Propargyl alcohol is probably metabolised to propargyl aldehyde, which causes marked inhibition of acetaldehyde dehydrogenase and is thought to be responsible for the liver damage which occurs on administration of pargyline (N-methyl-N-propargyl benzylamine), an aminooxidase inhibitor (DeMaster and Nagasawa, 1978; DeMaster et al. 1982, 1986).

7.2 Acute and subacute toxicity

The following LD_{50} values were determined after acute oral and intraperitonal administration:

Table 1. LD_{50} values for different species

Species	Route of administration	LD_{50}
Mouse	oral	50 mg/kg
Mouse	i.p.	45 mg/kg
Rat	oral	between 20 and 110 mg/kg
Rabbit	oral	> 19 < 39 mg/kg
Guinea-pig	oral	> 39 < 97 mg/kg
Cat	oral	> 10 < 19 mg/kg

For further information see Table 2.

After oral and intraperitoneal administration, the following effects were seen:

Mouse, rat: Excitation, accelerated breathing and lying on the stomach. At autopsy, blood was found in the gut contents, focal bleeding was seen in the lungs, and there was also bleeding in the pancreas and thymus, congestion of the liver and lungs, and liver damage (BASF, 1963; Archer, 1985).

Table 2 . Acute toxicity of propargyl alcohol

Species	Number of animals/dose	Sex	Route of exposure	Observation period (days)	No effect level (mg/kg bw)	LD_{50}/LC_{50} (95% confidence limits)	References
Mouse	–	–	oral	–	–	50 ± 3.1 mg/kg bw	Stasenkova and Kochetkova, 1966
Mouse	–	♂, ♀	i.p.	7	–	46.5 µl/kg bw $\hat{=}$ 45.2 mg/kg bw (37.3–59.5 µl/kg bw $\hat{=}$ 36.2–57.8 mg/kg bw)	BASF, 1963
Rat (Sprague-Dawley)	–	♂	oral	–	–	93 mg/kg bw (58–150 mg/kg bw)	Vernot et al., 1977
Rat (Sprague-Dawley)	4	♂	oral	2	80	110 mg/kg bw (100–120 mg/kg bw)	Archer, 1985
Rat (Sprague-Dawley)	–	♀	oral	–	–	54 mg/kg bw (37–78 mg/kg bw)	Vernot et al., 1977
Rat (Sprague-Dawley)	4	♀	oral	2	50	55 mg/kg bw (50–60 mg/kg bw)	Archer, 1985
Rat	–	–	oral	–	–	20–50 mg/kg bw	Dow, 1982

Rat	—	♂, ♀	oral	7	—	58 µl/kg bw $\hat{=}$ 56.4 mg/kg bw (48.0–70.0 µl/kg bw $\hat{=}$ 46.6–68.0 mg/kg bw)	BASF, 1963
Rat	—	—	oral	—	—	70 mg/kg bw	General Aniline and Film Corp., 1972
Rat (Sprague-Dawley)	5	♂	inhalation (1 hour)	—	—	1200 ppm (1180–1220 ppm)	Vernot et al., 1977
Rat (Sprague-Dawley)	5	♀	inhalation (1 hour)	—	—	1040 ppm (970–1120 ppm)	Vernot et al., 1977
Rabbit	—	—	oral	—	—	>0.02 <0.04 ml/kg bw $\hat{=}$ >19<39 mg/kg bw	BASF, 1987
Rabbit (New Zealand)	3	♀	dermal (24 hours)	—	—	88 mg/kg bw	Vernot et al., 1977
Rabbit	—	—	dermal	—	—	ca. 16 mg/kg bw	Dow, 1982
Guinea-pig	—	—	oral	—	—	>0.04 <0.1 ml/kg bw $\hat{=}$ >39 <97 mg/kg bw	BASF, 1987
Guinea-pig	—	—	oral	—	—	60 mg/kg bw	General Aniline and Film Corp., 1982
Cat	—	—	oral	—	—	>0.01 <0.02 ml/kg bw $\hat{=}$ >10 <19 mg/kg bw	BASF, 1987

– no information

Guinea-pig: Apathy, atonia, damage to the liver and kidneys (no further details given; BASF, 1987).

Rabbit: Accelerated breathing, diarrhoea, apathy, atonia, lying on the side, tonic spasms, paresis, protein in the urine, erythrocytes and kidney epithelia in urinary sediment, hyperaemia of the viscera and bleeding of the stomach, intestines and musculature (BASF, 1987; Tietze, 1926).

Cat: Bleeding in the thymus and abdominal cavity, defective gastric mucosa, damage to the liver and kidneys (no further details given; BASF, 1987).

A single dermal application of 194 mg/kg for 24 hours was fatal to three rabbits (BASF, 1963).

An LD_{50} value of 88 mg/kg body weight was determined in rabbits after occlusive application of propargyl alcohol to clipped skin for 24 hours (Vernot et al., 1977).

In a further study on rabbits, the LD_{50} value for undiluted propargyl alcohol was found to be about 16 mg/kg after percutaneous administration (no further details). The neat liquid caused hyperaemia with oedema formation and superficial necrosis. A 10% solution caused slight hyperaemia and oedema formation, and long-term exposure at this concentration also caused some deaths (no further details). A 1% solution had no effect (Dow, 1982).

Occlusive application of propargyl alcohol at doses of 0.05 ml/kg ($\overset{\wedge}{=}$48.6 mg/kg), 0.1 ml/kg ($\overset{\wedge}{=}$97.2 mg/kg) or 0.2 ml/kg ($\overset{\wedge}{=}$194.3 mg/kg) to the backs of rabbits (three per group) for 24 hours was fatal to all the animals at the higher doses, either during or shortly after exposure. Two of the three rabbits exposed to 0.05 ml/kg survived. Local tissue necrosis of variable severity was seen, as well as apathy and diarrhoea. Autopsy of the animals in the highest dose group revealed bleeding in the stomach and hyperaemia of the intestines. The observation period was 3 weeks (BASF, 1987).

In a dermal study on Sprague-Dawley rats (five animals/group) a single dose of 2 ml propargyl alcohol was applied for 1, 3 or 10 minutes to the clipped skin of the abdomen. The application area was roughly 10% of the surface area of the body. After treatment, the skin was washed with polyethylene glycol 400 and dried with cellulose. All of the animals that were exposed for 3 or 10 minutes died within a few hours of exposure, while there were no deaths on exposure for 1 minute. Symptoms of toxicity included apathy and irregular breathing. In the animals which were exposed for 10 minutes, necrosis and bleeding were seen at the application site, as well as bleeding in the thymus and jejunum (BASF, 1987).

A rabbit died $2^1/_2$ hours after a subcutanous injection of 200 µl propargyl alcohol/kg ($\hat{=}$ 194.3 mg/kg). A second rabbit given 39 µl/kg ($\hat{=}$ 37 mg/kg) died within $6^1/_2$ hours. This rabbit had tolerated 19 µl/kg ($\hat{=}$ 19 mg/kg) subccutaneously on the previous day without adverse effects (Tietze, 1926).

In a preliminary industrial toxicology study, ten mice, ten rats, four guinea-pigs, two rabbits and one cat all exposed for 1 hour to propargyl alcohol vapour at a concentration of ca. 1300 ppm showed slight irritation of the mucous membranes. Apathy, vomiting and lying on the side were also seen in the cat, which died 2 days after exposure. Clinical-chemical studies revealed functional disturbances in the liver and kidneys of the cat and the rabbits. In this study, three of the ten mice and one of the ten rats died after 1–3 days, while all four guinea-pigs and the rabbits survived (BASF, 1965).

In an inhalation-risk test, exposure for 3 minutes to an atmosphere saturated with propargyl alcohol (at 20° C) caused six out of twelve rats to die, while exposures of 10 minutes or longer caused the deaths of all of the exposed animals (six animals per exposure time). Most of the animals died a few hours after the beginning of the study, although some survived for 1–2 days. Symptoms of acute toxicity included flight behaviour at the beginning of exposure, irritation of the mucous membranes, marked pallor of the ears and paws and shortness of breath. Macroscopic examination revealed isolated bleeding in the gastro-intestinal region (BASF, 1963).

Similar results were obtained in a further study. Inhalation exposure for 6 minutes to an atmosphere saturated with propargyl alcohol led to the deaths of two out of three rats, while a 12-minute exposure caused all the animals to die (Dow, 1982).

In the mouse, a 2-hour exposure to propargyl alcohol at a concentration of 2 mg/l ($\hat{=}$ 874 ppm) led to the deaths of all the exposed animals (no further details; Stasenkova and Kochetkova, 1966).

Groups of ten male and ten female rats received daily doses of 0, 5, 15 or 45 mg propargyl alcohol/kg in aqueous solution by stomach tube for 4 weeks. At 5 mg/kg, an increase in liver and kidney weights occurred which did not correlate with any histological findings. From 15 mg/kg, signs of hypochromic anaemia were recognizable. A dose of 45 mg/kg retarded body-weight gain and increased alanine-aminotransferase, alkaline phosphatase and glutamate dehydrogenase activities in male rats, as well as histologically-confirmed liver cell damage. In a subsequent 4-week study with doses of 50 or 60 mg/kg, marked symptoms of toxicity occurred (apathy, atonia, bloody salivation) and one of the 15 treated rats died. At this dose level, the activity of γ-glutamyl transferase was markedly increased. The authors concluded that 50 or 60 mg/kg was the maximum tolerated dose and 5 mg/kg was the threshold dose (Bayer, 1984).

No treatment-related mortality was seen in rabbits on oral administration of propargyl alcohol, twenty times (five times per week), at a dose of 0.01 ml/kg ($\hat{=}$ 9.7 mg/kg). However, a dose of 0.02 ml/kg ($\hat{=}$ 19.4 mg/kg) caused all the animals to die after 9–23 days of treatment. Dilation of the peripheral vessels, and signs of lung congestion and exudation were found in the dead animals, as well as bleeding in the gastro-intestinal tract and heart muscle. Histological examination revealed slight liver and kidney damage (BASF, 1987).

Two cats given 0.01 ml/kg ($\hat{=}$ 9.7 mg/kg) propargyl alcohol orally, five times a week, died on days 16 and 17 of treatment. Toxicity was characterized by vomitting, loss of appetite and weight loss; in one of the animals, liver function was considerably disturbed. Histological examination revealed liver and kidney damage (BASF, 1987).

Inhalation of ca. 1300 ppm (static study, nominal concentration) for 1 hour daily for 5 days by mice, rats, guinea-pigs, rabbits and cats led to the findings which are presented in Table 2. The observation period for the surviving animals was 3 weeks. Body-weight gain in these animals was normal. Clinical examination of the blood (including clotting), urine, liver and kidneys revealed no adverse effects (BASF, 1965).

7.3   Skin and mucous membrane effects

A 1-minute application of undiluted propargyl alcohol (no details of dose) to the backs of rabbits caused very slight oedema formation within 24 hours. Slight necrosis was seen 8 days after application. 5- or 15-minute exposures resulted in very slight oedema formation and bleeding of the skin. Eight days after application, severe necrosis and anaemia were evident. The irritant effect of a 20-hour application of the undiluted product could not be determined, because the rabbits died after 4 hours (BASF, 1963).

One hour after instillation of 50µl undiluted propargyl alcohol into the conjunctival sacs of rabbits, slight reddening of the mucous membranes, pronounced oedema formation and slight clouding of the cornea were seen. These effects remained almost unchanged during the first days of the observation period. Eight days after application, a scar developed on the upper lid. The reddening of the mucous membranes and the oedema had not cleared up by then (BASF, 1963).

In a further study on eye irritation in rabbits, the instillation of undiluted propargyl alcohol into the conjunctival sac produced clear signs of pain, irritation and permanent corneal damage (no further details). A 10% solution caused slight irritation, which cleared up within a few days. No irritation was evident with a 1% solution (Dow, 1982).

7.4 Sensitization

A citation in the literature describes propargyl alcohol as non-sensitizing (no further details; General Aniline and Film Corporation, 1982).

7.5 Subchronic and chronic toxicity

In a preliminary study in mice, rats, guinea-pigs, rabbits and cats, a concentration of ca. 100 ppm propargyl alcohol (static study, nominal concentration, 6 hours daily, 5 times/week, 1–75 days of treatment) led to irritation of the mucous membranes. Detailed results are presented in Table 3 (BASF, 1987).

In further studies involving subchronic inhalation exposure (treatment for 59 days, total study duration 89 days), 12 male and 12 female rats were exposed to 80 ppm propargyl alcohol in the atmosphere (7 hours/day, 5 days/week). Twelve rats of each sex served as the controls. On the first day of the study, propargyl alcohol caused irritation of the mucous membranes and lethargic behaviour. These symptoms were no longer apparent during further exposure. Increased liver weight was seen in male rats, while in the females both liver and kidney weights were increased. Histological examination revealed degenerative damage to the liver and kidneys, which was more marked in the females (Dow, 1982).

In rabbits, there were no indications of systemic toxicity on dermal application of 1, 3 or 10 mg propargyl alcohol/kg/day for 63 days or 20 mg/kg/day for 28 days. Parameters studied included body weight, haematology and histopathology. The study gave no details of local effects (General Aniline and Film Corporation, 1982).

Table 3. Subacute inhalation toxicity of propargyl alcohol (ca. 1300 ppm for 1 hour/day for 5 days, static study, nominal concentration; BASF, 1965)

Species	Dead/exposed animals	Findings
Mouse	7/10 (after 2–3 exposures)	Irritation of the mucous membranes dead animals: suspected liver damage
Rat	4/10 (after 3–4 exposures)	Irritation of the mucous membranes dead animals: liver damage (jaundice) No findings at autopsy
Guinea-pig	0/4	Irritation of the mucous membranes
Rabbit	1/2 (6 days after the 5th exposure)	Irritation of the mucous membranes dead animals: hydrothorax, fatty liver No findings at autopsy
Cat	1/1 (after the 2nd exposure)	Irritation of the mucous membranes, lying prone, tonic clonic spasms, opisthotonos Autopsy: petechial bleeding in various organs, surface of the liver spotted, bloody mucus in the stomach, blood in the abdominal cavity, histologically toxic dystrophy of the liver

7.6 Genotoxicity

In *Salmonella typhimurium* his D3052 without metabolic activation, propargyl alcohol had a weak mutagenic effect (15 revertants/μmol) compared with propargyl aldehyde (1370 revertants/μmol). Metabolic activation did not increase the activity (Basu and Marnett, 1984).

Propargyl alcohol was not mutagenic in *Salmonella thypimurium* strains TA 98, TA 100, TA 1535, TA 1537 or TA 1538 at doses of 4-2500 μg/plate, with or without metabolic activation. At high concentrations, the product was cytotoxic (BASF, 1979).

Table 4. Subacute inhalation toxicity of propargyl alcohol (ca. 100 ppm 6 hours/day, 5 days/week, static study, nominal concentration; BASF, 1987)

Species	Number of exposures	Dead/exposed animals	Findings
Mouse	1–53	38/60	Irritation of the mucous membranes, slight liver damage
Rat	1–75	13/30	Irritation of the mucous membranes
Guinea-pig	21–75	2/16	Irritation of the mucous membranes
Rabbit	45–75	2/3	Irritation of the mucous membranes
Cat	29–43	3/3	Irritation of the mucous membranes, slight liver damage, severe weight loss

7.7   Carcinogenicity
No information available.

7.8   Reproductive toxicity
No information available.

7.9   Effects on the immune system
No information available.

7.10 Neurotoxicity
No information available.

7.11 Other effects
No information available.

8.   Experience in humans

No information available.

9.   Threshold limit values

MAK-value: 2 ppm (5 mg/m^3; DFG, 1969)
TLV-value: 1 ppm (2 mg/m^3; ACGIH, 1986)

References

ACGIH (American Conference of Governmental Industrial Hygienists Inc.)
Documentation of the Threshold Limit Values and Biological Exposure Indices
5th Edition
Cincinnati, Ohio (1986)

Archer, T.E.
Acute oral toxicity as LD$_{50}$ (mg/kg) of propargyl alcohol to male and female rats
J. Environ. Sci. Health, B20, 593–596 (1985)

BASF AG
Unpublished report no. XIII 62 of 26.3.1963

BASF AG
Subakute Inhalationstoxizität von Propargylalkohol
Unpublished report of 18.5.1965

BASF AG
Unpublished report no. XVII 111 of 14.4.1987

BASF AG
Bericht über die Prüfung von Propin-1-ol-3 im Ames-Test
Unpublished report of 12.12.1979

BASF AG
Communication of 18.2.1987

Basu, A.K., Marnett, L.J.
Molecular requirements for the mutagenicity of malondialdehyde and related acroleins
Cancer Res., 44, 2848–2854 (1984)

Bayer AG
Unpublished report no. 12653 (1984)

Clayton, G.D., Clayton, F.E. (eds.)
Patty's Industrial Hygiene and Toxicology
3rd Edition, volume 2c
John Wiley, New York (1982)

DeMaster, E.G., Nagasawa, H.T.
Inhibition of aldehyde dehydrogenase by propiolaldehyde, a possible
metabolite of pargyline
Res. Commun. Chem. Pathol. Pharmacol., 21, 497–505 (1978)

DeMaster, E.G., Sumner, H.W., Kaplan, E., Shirota, F.N., Nagasawa, H.T.
Pargyline-induced hepatotoxicity: possible mediation by the reactive
metabolite, propiolaldehyde
Toxicol. Appl. Pharmacol., 65, 390–401 (1982)

DeMaster, E.G., Shirota, F.N., Nagasawa, H.T.
Role of propiolaldehyde and other metabolites in the pargyline
inhibition of rat liver aldehyde dehydrogenase
Biochem. Pharmacol., 35, 1481–1489 (1986)

DFG (Deutsche Forschungsgemeinschaft)
Commission for the Investigation of Health Hazards of Chemical
Compounds in the Work Area. Report No. V. Maximum
Concentrations of Dangerous Substances in the Workplace 1968
(MAK Values)
Publishing House of DFG, 1969

The Dow Chemical Company
Unpublished, cited in: Clayton and Clayton (1982)

General Aniline and Film Corporation
Cited in: Clayton and Clayton (1982)

Falbe, J., Bahrmann, H., Lipps, W., Grübler, P.
Ullmann's Encyclopedia of Industrial Chemistry
5th Edition, volume A1, 298 (1985)
VCH Verlagsgesellschaft, Weinheim

Hommel, G. (ed.)
Handbuch der gefährlichen Güter
Data sheet 970
Springer, Berlin Heidelberg New York (1985)

Stasenkova, K.P., Kochetkova, T.A.
Toxicological characteristics of propargyl alcohol
Toksikol. Novykh. Prom. Khim. Veshchestv., 8, 97–111 (1966)
see Chemical Abstracts 67, 89293b (1967)

Tietze, K.
Wirkung von Acetylencarbonsäure (Propargylsäure)
Medizin. Klinik, No. 48, 1843–1845 (1926)

Vernot, E.H., MacEwen, J.D., Haun, C.C., Kinkead, E.R.
Acute toxicity and skin corrosion data for some organic and inorganic
compounds and aqueous solutions
Toxicol. Appl. Pharmacol., 42, 417–423 (1977)

Diethanolamine

1. Summary and assessment

The toxicity findings published in the literature up until 1981 have been reported and evaluated by the MAK Commission in their publication on toxicity and industrial medicine (Henschler, 1981).

These indicate that the substance is of moderate acute toxicity (LD_{50} rats, oral, between 780 and 3.540 mg/kg) and causes severe irritation to the skin and eyes. According to abstracts describing sub-chronic tests in rats (a feeding study and an inhalation study, both over 3 months), the oral "no-effect-level" appears to lie between 20 and 90 mg/kg body weight, whilst a "no-effect-level" for inhalation exposure cannot be determined. Even a concentration of 6 ppm produces marked symptoms of toxicity and a few deaths.

The difficulty with diethanolamine lies in the fact that it is nitrosatable (expecially in acidic conditions), thus forming N-nitrosodiethanolamine, a known carcinogen in rats and hamsters.

The results of further investigations have been published since 1981:

Repeated dermal applications (twelve times) of 0.1 to 2.0 g/kg to rats and 0.2 to 3.0 g/kg to mice causes deaths at the higher doses. The lower doses produce chronic skin inflammation and, in the rats, microscopically-detectable kidney damage and necrosis of the seminiferous tubules.

The recognized local irritant effects on skin and eyes are confirmed by the new literature. According to tests, of which no further details were given, diethanolamine has no skin-sensitizing effect in guinea-pigs.

Thirteen-week subchronic studies in rats, involving administration in the drinking water or dermal application, resulted in dose-dependent microcytosis and non-regenerative anaemia, effects which are evident down to the lower doses (0.32 mg/ml in the drinking water, corresponding to ca. 30 mg/kg body weight). Other target organs include the kidneys and the central nervous system (demyelinisation). Analogous studies in mice resulted in changes to the liver and kidney, which occur down to the concentration of 0.63 mg/ml drinking water, corresponding to ca. 100 mg/kg body weight for males and ca. 140 mg/kg for females (lowest dose).

Diethanolamine shows no mutagenic or cell-transforming properties.

A screening test provides indications of a fetotoxic effect.

More than 50 cases have been described of neuroparalytic symptoms in dogs and cats after oral administration of a formulation against fleas. The formulation was a 53% aqueous solution of diethanolamine (individual daily dose 44 mg/kg).

The possibility of N-nitrosodiethanolamine-formation in rats after dermal application of diethanolamine and simultaneous oral administration of high levels of nitrite must be taken into consideration.

Epidemiological studies on people who work with cutting oils containing nitrite and diethanolamine have indicated no increase in the mortality rate or in the number of cancer deaths.

In the USA, a threshold limit value of 3 ppm≈13 mg/m^3 in the work place is in force for diethanolamine. However, this is not sufficiently justified.

The following additional tests are being performed on behalf of BG-Chemie:
– 90-day inhalation test (rats), including a neurotoxicity test
– Sensitization study in guinea-pigs
– Teratogenicity/embryotoxicity inhalation study in rats.

A final evaluation cannot be undertaken until the studies which are still outstanding have been completed.

2.   Name of substance

2.1   Usual name   Diethanolamine
2.2   IUPAC-name   Bis-(2-hydroxyethyl)amine
2.3   CAS-No.   111-42-2

3.   Synonyms, common and trade names

2,2′-Aminodiethanol
N,N-Diethanolamine
Diethylolamine
2,2′-Dihydroxy-diethylamine
β,β′-Dihydroxy-diethylamine
Di-(2-hydroxyethyl)amine
Diolamine
2,2′-Iminobisethanol
2,2′-Iminodiethanol
DEA

4.   Structural and molecular formulae

4.1   Structural formula

$$HO-CH_2-CH_2 \diagdown$$
$$\qquad\qquad\qquad NH$$
$$HO-CH_2-CH_2 \diagup$$

4.2   Molecular formula $C_4H_{11}NO_2$

5.   Physical and chemical properties

5.1   Molecular mass, g/mol   105.14

5.2   Melting point, °C   28 (Ciba-Geigy, 1974)

5.3   Boiling point, °C   268–269 (Ciba-Geigy,
                                       1974)

5.4   Vapour pressure, hPa   <0.013 (at 20 °C;
                                       BASF, 1986)
                                     6 (at 138 °C; BASF, 1986)

5.5   Density, g/cm^3 1.097 (at 20 °C;
                                       Ciba-Geigy, 1974)

5.6   Solubility in water   fully miscible at > 28 °C (BASF,
                                       1986)

5.7   Solubility in organic solvents 4.2% in benzene,
                                       0.8% in ether,
                                       miscible with acetone
                                       and methanol,
                                       <0.1% in carbon
                                       tetrachloride,
                                       <0.1% in n-heptane
                                       (Windholz, 1983)

5.8   Solubility in fat   No information available.

5.9   pH-value   11 (at 53 g/l; BASF, 1986)

5.10 Conversion factor   1 ppm $\hat{=}$ 4.36 mg/m^3
                                     1 mg/m^3 $\hat{=}$ 0.23 ppm
                                     (at 25 °C and 1013 hPa)

6.   Uses

Intermediate in the manufacture of dyes, optical brighteners, rubber chemicals, wetting agents and plasticizers; additive for agrochemicals, cosmetics, pharmaceuticals, cutting and drilling oils, cleaning and polishing agents, detergents and textile chemicals; constituent of lubricants and surface-active preparations; corrosion inhibitor in cooling lubricants for metal-cutting (Windholz, 1983).

7.   Experimental results

Like other secondary amines, diethanolamine may be contaminated with the corresponding nitrosamine, N-nitroso-diethanolamine (NDEIA; Spiegelhalder et al., 1978); concentrations ranging from 5 to 1460 µg/kg have been measured (Sommer et al., 1988). NDEIA is a potent chemical carcinogen in animal experiments (Preussmann et al., 1982).

7.1   Toxicokinetics and metabolism
No information available.

7.2   Acute and subacute toxicity
Diethanolamine in ethanol was applied dermally (between the shoulder blades) to F-344 rats and B6C3F1 mice, 12 times within 16 days. Doses for rats were between 0.1 and 2.0 g/kg and for mice between 0.2 and 3.0 g/kg (12 doses each, concentrations not specified). The highest doses were lethal to rats and mice. At doses of 0.5 g/kg and above (concentrations not specified), chronic inflammation, ulceration and acanthosis were seen in rats at the application site. Mice showed the same symptoms at concentrations of 1.25 g/kg and above (a figure of 1.25 mg/kg is given in the publication, but this is obviously an error). Slight acanthosis was also seen in mice in the lowest dose group. Microscopically detectable necroses of the renal and seminiferous tubules also occurred in rats receiving high doses. The authors concluded that rats are more sensitive to diethanolamine than mice and that systemic poisoning by dermal application is possible (Melnick et al., 1988).

7.3   Skin and mucous membrane effects
Diethanolamine (purity 98%) was tested for irritant effects on the skin and eyes of rabbits, in accordance with the French guidelines (no further details). The irritant effect was measured on intact and abraded skin (number of animals and exposure time not given). The primary irritation index (I.I.P.) for diethanolamine was 2.6 (out of a maximum of 8.0) and was evaluated as moderate (compared with monoethanolamine, I.I.P. 7.0, severe; and triethanolamine, I.I.P. 1.5, slight). The irritant effect was more severe on abraded skin than on

intact skin. On the latter, after 72 hours, the erythema was worsening whilst the oedema was abating (Dutertre-Catella et al., 1982).

In rabbits' eyes, the irritation index (I.I.O.) for diethanolamine was ≥50 (from a maximum of 110) after 24 hours, 56 after 48 hours, 52 after 72 hours, 45 after 96 hours and 41 after 7 days. The overall irritant effect was designated as severe. For comparison, the maximum irritation index for monoethanolamine was ≥96 (after 96 hours and 7 days) and for triethanolamine was 0 (at all evaluation times; Dutertre-Catella et al., 1982).

7.4   Sensitization

Diethanolamine was tested, along with ten other chemicals, for its sensitizing effect on guinea-pig skin (method and number of animals used not specified). The product was not sensitizing (Kharchenko and Ivanova, 1980).

7.5   Subchronic and chronic toxicity

In a study of the subchronic toxicity of diethanolamine (purity ca. 97%), groups of ten male and ten female Fischer-344 rats (weight 106–176 g) received 20, 50, 100, 200 or 400 mg/kg body weight as an aqueous solution by stomach tube for 13 weeks. At 100 mg/kg or more, seven out of ten males died before the end of the experiment, or had to be killed due to their moribund condition. At 200 mg/kg or more, the equivalent number of females that died or were killed was two out of ten. Compared to the control group, body weight gain was retarded in the males by 11% (50 mg/kg), 21% (100 mg/kg), 23% (200 mg/kg) or 51% (400 mg/kg) and in the females by 9% (100 mg/kg), 27% (200 mg/kg) or 75% (400 mg/kg). Symptoms observed were emaciation from week 6 (males) or week 10 (females) and tremors in one animal in weeks 12 and 13. No treatment-related effects were noted on autopsy or, initially, on histological examination. However, during quality control, mineral deposition was found in the kidneys of eight out of ten females in the 200 and 400 mg/kg dose groups, and hyperplasia and hyperkeratosis of the stomach were evident in four out of ten males of the 400 mg/kg group. No other parameters were investigated. On the basis of these findings, the suggested dose levels for a 2-year study were 20 and 50 mg/kg for male rats and 50 and 100 mg/kg for female rats (GSRI, 1980).

An analogous study was carried out with groups of ten male and ten female B6C3F1 mice (weight 18–28 g) at doses of 50, 100, 200, 400 or 800 mg/kg body weight. Before the end of the study, two males in the 800 mg/kg group and one female in the 100 mg/kg group died. Body-weight gain of male rats was impaired by 40% (200 mg/kg), 28% (400 mg/kg) or 44% (800 mg/kg), while the females showed a gain in weight of between 20 and 47%, independent of the dose. Alopecia occurred in the males from 200 mg/kg and in the females from 100 mg/kg. Autopsy revealed no treatment-related effects. Again, there were no findings in the initial histological examination, but quality control revealed effects on the kidneys of male mice in the 800 mg/kg group (increased and abnormal mitoses in the kidney cortex, casts and eosinophilic material in the lumina of the tubules). In one female in this dose group, such effects were minimal. No other parameters were investigated. In view of these findings, levels of 200 and 400 mg/kg for male mice and 400 and 800 mg/kg for female mice were suggested for a 2-year study (GSRI, 1980).

In a further study, groups of ten male and ten female Fischer-344 rats (weight 66–100 g) were exposed to diethanolamine (purity >99%) in the drinking water for 13 weeks. The doses were, for the males, 0.32, 0.63, 1.25, 2.5 or 5 mg/ml water (corresponding to 28.3, 55, 109, 233.2 or 487.5 mg/kg body weight), and for the females, 0.16, 0.32, 0.63, 1.25 or 2.5 mg/ml water (corresponding to 15, 36, 64, 141.4 and 248.6 mg/kg body weight). One rat in the 5 mg/ml group died on day 54 of the study and a second from the same group had to be killed on day 71 due to its moribund condition. Observed symptoms included tremors, emaciation, abnormal posture and ruffled fur, effects which were most pronounced in the highest two dose groups. Haematological examination of both sexes revealed a dose-dependent reduction in haemoglobin level, erythrocyte count, haematocrit level, average erythrocyte volume and average corpuscular haemoglobin content ($p \leq 0.05$ and 0.01) at doses down to 0.32 mg/ml (corresponding to 28 mg/kg body weight in the males and 36 mg/kg body weight in the females). No compensatory rise in reticulocytes occurred. Notable findings in the clinical-chemical investigations included a dose-dependent increase in blood urea ($p \leq 0.05$ and 0.01) and in bile acids ($p \leq 0.05$ and 0.01). Autopsy revealed no treatment-related effects. A dose-dependent increase in the relative liver weights was seen ($p \leq 0.01$) down to 0.63 mg/ml (corresponding to 55 mg/kg body weight) in male rats, and down to 0.16 mg/ml (corresponding to 15 mg/kg body weight) in female rats. There was also a dose-dependent increase in the relative kidney weights ($p \leq 0.01$) from 0.32 mg/ml (corresponding to 28 mg/kg body weight) in males and from 0.16 mg/ml (corresponding to 15 mg/kg body weight) in females (in both cases the lowest dose). Histological examination revealed mainly nephropathy and mineral deposition in the kidney tubules of the females, down to the lowest dose (0.16 mg/ml, corresponding to 15 mg/kg body weight). Furthermore, demyelinisation of the medullary sheaths in the brain and spinal cord was observed in the females up to a dose of 0.63 mg/ml (corresponding to 64 mg/kg body weight). Other findings included disturbances in cell division of the spermatocytes with hypospermia in the epididymides, atrophy of the seminal vesicles, cytosplasmic vacuolisation of the adrenal cortex, lymphocyte depletion in the thymus, and hyperplasia of alveolar macrophages in the lungs. These findings were generally only observed at the higher doses (from 1.25 mg/ml; Battelle, 1988a).

A second drinking-water study on diethanolamine (purity >99%) was carried out with groups of ten male and ten female B6C3F1 mice (weight 18.5–26.9 g) for 13 weeks. The doses used were 0.63, 1.25, 2.50, 5.0 or 10.0 mg/ml water, corresponding to 103.6, 178.0, 422.4, 806.5 or 1673.8 mg/kg body weight respectively for males and 142.3, 346.8, 883.6, 1153.8 or 2128.2 mg/kg body weight respectively for females. All the mice in the 5 and 10 mg/ml groups, as well as three of the ten females in the 2.5 mg/ml group, died before the end of the experiment. Water intake was decreased at the two highest doses (males −16.7 and −18.8% respectively; females −30.4 and −68.1% respectively). Body-weight gain was reduced in the 2.5 mg/ml dose group by 30.4% (males) and 45.4% (females), and in females of the 1.25 mg/ml group by 23.1%. Observed symptoms included emaciation, ruffled fur, abnormal posture and hypoactivity. No haematological studies were carried out. Clinical-chemical analysis revealed an increase in serum albumin (p ≤ 0.01) in both sexes at doses of 0.63 mg/ml or more, and an increase in alanine aminotransferase activity at 2.5 mg/ml (p ≤ 0.01) in the males and at 1.25 mg/ml or more (p ≤ 0.05 and 0.01) in the females. Sorbitol dehydrogenase activity was also increased (p ≤ 0.01) in males in the 2.5 mg/ml group. Autopsy of the mice killed at the end of the study period revealed no treatment-related effects. A dose-dependent increase in the relative liver weight (p ≤ 0.01) was recorded from 0.63 mg/ml in both sexes, as well as an increase in the relative kidney weight (p ≤ 0.01) from 1.25 mg/ml in the males and from 2.5 mg/ml in the females. An increase in the relative heart weight (p ≤ 0.01) was seen in male mice of the 2.5 mg/ml group and in females in the 1.25 and 2.5 mg/ml groups. Histologically, degeneration of the heart muscle was seen in a few animals of the 2.5 mg/ml group. Liver cell damage was observed in all treated mice, and liver cell necrosis occurred in all dose groups except the 0.63 mg/ml group. In addition, kidney damage occurred in males from 1.25 mg/ml (Batelle, 1988b).

The dermal toxicity of diethanolamine (purity >99%) was investigated in a 13-week study using groups of ten male and ten female Fischer 344-rats (71.0–113.52 g). The doses used were 32, 63, 125, 250 or 500 mg/kg body weight. A solution of diethanolamine in 95% ethanol (USP) was applied to the clipped dorsal skin at concentrations of 3.75, 7.5, 15, 30 or 60% diethanolamine. In the highest dose group (500 mg/kg), one of the ten males died in the 9th week and two of the ten females were killed in the 10th week (because of their moribund condition). Body-weight gain of the males of the 250 and 500 mg/kg groups was reduced by 21 and 45.8% respectively, while that of the females was reduced at doses of 63 mg/kg or more by 11.8, 15.7, 25.2 and 48%, respectively. Locally, skin irritation and crust formation were observed, which increased with increasing dose and concentration. Two females in the highest dose group showed severe emaciation. Haematological examination produced similar results to those in the drinking water study. A significant decrease in haemoglobin concentration, erythrocyte count and haematocrit level occurred dose-dependently in male rats from concentrations of 125, 250 and 63 mg/kg respectively, and in female rats from 32 mg/kg (all parameters $p \leq 0.01$). No compensatory reticulocytosis was seen. Clinical-chemical investigation revealed increased blood urea levels in both sexes from 250 mg/kg ($p \leq 0.05$ and 0.01), and increased alanine aminotransferase activity in males from 125 mg/kg ($p \leq 0.05$) and in females at 500 mg/kg ($p \leq 0.01$). Autopsy revealed marked crust formation and red or brown staining of the skin at the application site, effects which increased with increasing dose and concentration. There were dose-dependent increases in the relative liver weight (in males from 125 mg/kg, $p \leq 0.01$; in females from 32 mg/kg, $p \leq 0.01$), the relative kidney weight (in males and females from 32 mg/kg, $p \leq 0.01$) and the relative testis weight (from 250 mg/kg, $p \leq 0.01$). Histological examination revealed dose- and concentration-dependent ulceration and crusting of the skin, coagulation necrosis and chronic inflammation with proliferation or slight hyperkeratosis at the lower doses. Effects on the kidney tubules included necroses, mineral deposition, protein casts, chronic inflammation of the interstitium of the kidney cortex and hyperplasia of the transitional epithelium of the renal calyces. The females were more severely affected than the males. Demyelinisation of the medulla oblongata also occurred. The liver was apparently without treatment-related effects. When both local and systemic effects were considered, a no-effect-level of 32 mg/kg was derived for male rats, while in females a no-effect-level could not be established (Battelle, 1988c).

An analogous dermal study was carried out with groups of ten male and ten female B6C3F1 mice (weight 17.5–24.7 g) for 13 weeks. The doses used were 80, 160, 320, 630 or 1250 mg/kg (no concentrations were specified, but it can be assumed that they were relatively high, as in the rat study). Two males of the 1250 mg/kg group had to be removed from the study in the 2nd and 9th week because of their moribund condition, and four females of the same dose group died or had to be killed in the 2nd or 3rd week. Locally, skin irritation with crust formation and skin thickening occurred, as well as staining of the hair, in the mice given 630 and 1250 mg/kg. No symptoms of toxicity were seen as a result of absorption. Body-weight gain was retarded by 24% in males of the highest dose group (1250 mg/kg), while the other mice were not affected. No haematological investigations were carried out. Clinical-chemical studies showed an increase in alanine aminotransferase activity ($p \leq 0.05$ and 0.01) in males at doses of 320 mg/kg or more, an effect which was observed in the females only at the highest dose (1250 mg/kg, $p \leq 0.01$). An increase in sorbitol dehydrogenase activity was also seen in males from 320 mg/kg ($p \leq 0.05$ and 0.01). Autopsy revealed local incrustation, red-brown staining of the skin and ulceration of the epidermis, seen in males of the upper two dose groups (1250 and 630 mg/kg) and in females of the highest dose group (1250 mg/kg). The relative liver weight increased dose-dependently ($p \leq 0.01$) in males from 160 mg/kg and in females from 80 mg/kg. Likewise, the relative kidney weight increased in males from 160 mg/kg and in females from 630 mg/kg ($p \leq 0.05$ and 0.01, respectively). In the 1250 mg/kg dose group, an increase in relative heart weight ($p \leq 0.01$) was seen in both sexes. Histologically, local effects included skin burns and ulceration, inflammation, hyperkeratosis and acanthosis, the latter down to 80 mg/kg would be seen. Liver cell damage was seen in all the treated males, but only at 160 mg/kg or more in the females. Furthermore, lymphocyte depletion was found in the spleen, thymus and lymph nodes (in males from 160 mg/kg, in females from 630 mg/kg). In females of the highest dose group (1250 mg/kg), necrosis of the kidney tubules, haemorrhages in the adrenals and dysplasia in the salivary glands were seen. Heart muscle degeneration was also evident in both sexes at the highest dose (1250 mg/kg). A no-effect-level for local and systemic effects could not be established. Based on these results, an upper dose of 320 mg/kg was suggested for a 2-year study (Battelle, 1988d).

7.6   Genotoxicity

7.6.1 In vitro

A study was carried out on *Salmonella typhimurium* strains TA 100, TA 1535, TA 1537 and TA 98 at doses of 0 (control), 33, 100, 333, 1000 and 3333μg/plate. The metabolising system was obtained from rats and hamsters (S9 mix from Aroclor 1254 pre-treated animals). Diethanolamine was not mutagenic in this study, either with or without metabolic activation (Haworth et al., 1983).

A further test on the possible mutagenic activity of diethanolamine (purity 99.7%) was carried out on *Salmonella typhimurium* strains TA 1535, TA 1537, TA 1538, TA 98 and TA 100, on *Escherichia coli* WP2 and WP2uvrA, and on *Saccharomyces cerevisiae* JD1. In addition, diethanolamine was tested in the rat liver cell lines RL_1 and RL_4 (epithelial-type cells) for chromosomal damage. The test was carried out with and without metabolic activation in the bacteria and yeasts. The doses used in the Salmonella/microsome tests and in the tests with *Escherichia coli* were 125, 250, 500, 1000, 2000 and 4000 μg/plate. In the studies on *Saccharomyces cerevisiae* and rat chromosomes, the doses used were not clearly specified. Diethanolamine was not mutagenic or clastogenic in these studies (Dean et al., 1985).

In a further study, diethanolamine was tested in the *Salmonella typhimurium* strains TA 1535 and TA 100 with and without metabolic activation (doses not specified). No point-mutagenic activity was seen (Hedenstedt, 1978).

Diethanolamine was also tested, together with a number of other chemicals, for point-mutagenic activity in the mouse lymphoma test in the cell line L5178Y $TK^{+/-}$. At least three tests without metabolic activation were carried out per chemical. If the results were negative, two or more tests with metabolic activation (Aroclor 1254-induced rat liver S9 mix) were subsequently carried out. Diethanolamine showed no mutagenic activity in this study (doses were not specified in the available abstract; Myhr et al., 1986).

These results have been confirmed by other authors (no further details; NTP, 1986).

Diethanolamine causes no increase in the incidences of sister chromatid exchange or chromosomal aberrations in Chinese hamster (CHO) cells at doses of 150–3010 µg/ml, either with or without metabolic activation (S9 mix from Aroclor 1254-induced rat liver; Loveday et al., 1989).

7.6.2 In vivo

No information available.

7.7 Carcinogenicity

Diethanolamine was tested *in vitro* in the cell transformation test on hamster embryo cells, at dose levels of 25, 50, 100, 200 and 500 µg/ml. Nine plates were evaluated at each dose level. Diethanolamine had no cell-transforming properties in this study, but was cytotoxic at concentrations of 200 and 500 µg/plate (Inoue et al., 1982).

7.8 Reproductive toxicity

In a screening test for reproductive toxicity, 50 CD-1 mice received 450 mg diethanolamine/kg in aqueous solution by stomach tube from days 6 to 15 of pregnancy. After birth, dams and offsprings were observed for 3 days. In this study, diethanolamine had no influence on maternal mortality, litter size or birth weight, but it did reduce the number of viable offsprings per litter, their survival rate and their weight gain (EHT, 1987).

No conventional studies with pure diethanolamine have been carried out. However, a hair dye formulation containing 2% diethanolamine has been tested in rats for prenatal toxicity. Twenty pregnant Charles-River CD rats each received 2 ml dye formulation (P-24)/kg ($\hat{=}$40 mg diethanolamine/kg) dermally on days 1, 4, 7, 10, 13, 16 and 19 of pregnancy. On day 20 the dams were killed, and the foetuses removed by Caesarean section. In comparison with the controls, the 2% diethanol-amine-containing dye preparation did not significantly affect the numbers of corpora lutea, implantation sites or live foetuses, or the sex distribution of the foetuses. The number of resorptions was unaffected and there was no significant difference with regard to soft tissue or skeletal anomalies. The most frequent anomaly in all groups, including the control group, was accessory ribs (Burnett et al., 1976).

7.9 Effects on the immune system
See Chapter 7.5.

7.10 Neurotoxicity
During 1980 and 1981, American veterinary surgeons in Florida reported more than 50 cases of neuroparalytic syndrome in cats and dogs. These animals had been treated with an oral flearepellant preparation for periods of between 2 days and 18 months (average 5 months). On analysis the product was found to contain a 53% aqueous solution of diethanolamine, providing an individual dose of 44 mg/kg body weight. The neuromuscular disturbances included tremors, stiffness of the hind legs, ataxia, paresis and lameness. Altogether, over 39 cases in dogs and 12 cases in cats were reported, with a mortality rate of 41%. One case in a dog was described at length (Sundlof and Mayhew, 1983).

7.11 Other effects
The effects of diethanolamine, together with a number of other chemicals, were investigated in isolated rat hepatocytes. The parameters for cytotoxicity were GOT and LDH release, cell viability after a 2-hour incubation period, urea synthesis, and the ATP-content after a 5-hour incubation period. Diethanolamine concentrations of 10, 1 and 0.1 mmol were used. After 2 hours of incubation, a concentration of 10 mmol (corresponding to 105 μg/ml) significantly increased ($p < 0.05$) the liberation of LDH, while the other parameters remained unchanged. The two lower concentrations were without effect. After a 5-hour incubation period, a significant reduction in urea synthesis occurred only at the highest concentration (10mmol). The other parameters remained unaffected (Story et al., 1983).

To investigate the formation of N-nitrosodiethanolamine *in vivo*, rats received 2000 ppm sodium nitrite in the drinking water for 6 days, a single dermal application of 100–400 mg diethanolamine/rat, and further nitrite treatment for another 5 days. N-Nitrosodiethanolamine excretion in the urine averaged 2.4 μg/animal (range 1–5 μg) after 100 mg diethanolamine, 35 μg/animal (range 15–114 μg) after 200 mg, 24 μg/animal (range 1–150 μg) after 300 mg and 20 μg/animal (range 2–85) after 400 mg. With relatively high doses of nitrites, the possibility of N-nitrosodiethanolamine formation after dermal application of diethanolamine must be considered (Preussmann et al., 1981).

8. Experience in humans

An epidemiological study investigating mortality and cancer morbidity was carried out on 219 people who were employed for at least one year (between 1950 and 1966) on machines where cutting oils containing amines (mostly diethanolamine and triethanolamine) and nitrites were used. Every person was followed up, with the aid of death registers and the cancer register, until the end of 1983. The difference between the observed and expected cases was then calculated by Poisson-distribution. No increase in the mortality rate was seen in the people exposed to cutting oils for 1 year or more or for 5 years or more. There was no significant difference between the observed and expected deaths due to cancer in either exposure group. No information was given on exposure levels. The authors considered the results to be negative, but an increased risk cannot be excluded because of the limited number of people studied (Järvholm et al., 1986).

A group of 32 patients who had been sensitized to ethylene diamine were investigated for possible cross-sensitization to a number of chemicals, including diethanolamine. The investigation was carried out in accordance with the Standard Patch Test Battery of GIRDCA (Gruppo Italiano di Ricerca sulle Dermattiti da Contatto e Ambientali). A 1% solution of diethanolamine in paraffin oil produced a positive reaction in one of the 32 patients (Balato et al., 1986).

9. Threshold limit values

Diethanolamine is included in section IIb of the 1980 list of MAK values; a MAK value for the chemicals in this category could not be set due to incomplete data being available (DFG, 1980).

The US TLV is 3 ppm $\hat{=}$ 13 mg/m^3 (ACGIH, 1989). However, this value is not fully justified, based as it is on the NOEL (20 mg/kg body weight) from a 3-month feeding study in rats and on the analogy to monoethanolamine (ACGIH, 1986).

References

ACGIH (American Conference of Governmental Industrial Hygienists) Threshold Limit Values and Biological Exposure Indices for 1989–1990 (TLVs)
Cincinnati, Ohio (1989)

ACGIH (American Conference of Governmental Industrial Hygienists,
Documentation of the Threshold Limit Values and Biological
Exposure Indices, Diethanolamine, 5th ed., p. 197 (1986)
Cincinnati, Ohio

Balato, N., Cusano, F., Lembo, G., Ayala, F.
Ethylenediamine dermatitis
Contact Dermatitis, 15, 263–265 (1986)

BASF AG
Basic product data, 24. 12. 1986

Battelle, Columbus, Ohio
The prechronic dosed water study of diethanolamine (CAS 111-42-2)
in Fischer 344 rats
Unpublished report, National Toxicology Program (1988 a)

Battelle, Columbus, Ohio
The prechronic dosed water study of diethanolamine (CAS 111-42-2)
in B6C3F1 mice
Unpublished report, National Toxicology Program (1988 b)

Battelle, Columbus, Ohio
The prechronic dermal study of diethanolamine (CAS 111-42-2) in
Fischer 344 rats
Unpublished report, National Toxicology Program (1988 c)

Battelle, Columbus, Ohio
The prechronic dermal study of diethanolamine (CAS 111-42-2) in
B6C3F1 mice
Unpublished report, National Toxicology Program (1988 d)

Burnett, C., Goldenthal, E.I., Harris, S.B., Wazeter, F.X., Strausburg,
J., Kapp, R., Voelker, R.
Teratology and percutaneous toxicity studies on hair dyes
J. Toxicol. Environ. Health, 1, 1027–1040 (1976)

Ciba-Geigy AG
Chemical data card No. 231, February 1974

Dean, B.J., Brooks, T.M., Hodson-Walker, G., Hutson, D.H.
Genetic toxicology testing of 41 industrial chemicals
Mutat. Res., 153, 57–77 (1985)

DFG (Deutsche Forschungsgemeinschaft)
Maximale Arbeitsplatzkonzentration 1980
Mitteilung XVI der Senatskommission zur Prüfung gesundheits-
schädlicher Arbeitsstoffe
Harald Boldt, Boppard (1980)

Dutertre-Catella, H., Nguyen, P.L., Ngoc Huyen V., Truhaut, R.
Etude comparative de l'agressivité cutanée et oculaire des éthan-
olamines (mono, di, tri et poly)
Arch. Mal. Prof., 43, 455–460 (1982)

EHT (Environmental Health and Testing Inc.), Cincinnati, Ohio
Screening of priority chemicals for reproductive hazards, monoeth-
anolamine, diethanolamine, triethanolamine; NTP 87–377, Final
Report (1987)

GSRI (Gulf South Research Institute), New Iberia, Louisiana 70560
Subchronic test of diethanolamine (C55174) in B6C3F1 mice and
Fischer 344 rats
Unpublished report for Tractor Jitco, Rockville, Maryland 20852
(1980)

Haworth, S., Lawlor, T., Mortelmans, K., Speck, W., Zeiger, E.
Salmonella mutagenicity test results for 250 chemicals
Environ. Mutagen., Suppl. 1, 3–142 (1983)

Hedenstedt, A.
Mutagenicity screening of industrial chemicals: seven aliphatic ami-
nes and one amide tested in the Salmonella/microsomal assay
Mutat. Res., 53, 198–199 (1978)

Henschler, D. (ed.)
Gesundheitsschädliche Arbeitsstoffe
Toxikologisch Arbeitsmedizinische Begründung von MAK-Werten
8th Issue 1981, Diethanolamine
VCH Verlagsgesellschaft mbH, Weinheim

Inoue, K., Sunakawa, T., Okamoto, K., Tanaka, Y.
Mutagenicity tests and in vitro transformation assays on triethanol-
amine
Mutat. Res., 101, 305–313 (1982)

Järvholm, B., Lavenius, B., Sällsten, G.
Cancer morbidity in workers exposed to cutting fluids containing
nitrites and amines
Brit. J. Ind. Med., 43, 563–565 (1986)

Kharchenko, T.F., Ivanova, T.P.
Hygienic evaluation of some bonding materials and chemical substances applied to skin
Gig. Tr. Prof. Zabol., 7, 63–64 (1980)
(English translation)

Loveday, K.S., Lugo, M.H., Resnick, M.A., Anderson, B.E., Zeiger, E.
Chromosome aberration and sister chromatid exchange test in Chinese hamster ovary cells in vitro: II. Results with 20 chemicals
Environ. Molec. Mutagen., 13, 60–94 (1989)

Melnick, R., Hejtmancik, M., Mezza, L., Ryan, M., Persing, R., Peters, A.
Comparative effects of triethanolamine (TEA) and diethanolamine (DEA) in short-term dermal studies
The Toxicologist, 8(1), 127 (1988)

Myhr, B.C., Bowers, L.R., Caspary, W.J.
Results from the testing of coded chemicals in the L5178Y TK$^{+/-}$ mouse lymphoma mutagenesis assay
Environ. Mutagen., 8, Suppl. 6, 58 (1986)

Preussmann, R., Spiegelhalder, B., Eisenbrand, G., Würtele, G., Hofmann, I.
Urinary excretion of N-nitrosodiethanolamine in rats following its epicutaneous and intratracheal administration and its formation *in vivo* following skin application of diethanolamine
Cancer Lett., 13, 227–231 (1981)

Preussmann, R., Habs, M., Habs, H., Schmähl, D.
Carcinogenicity of N-nitrosodiethanolamine in rats at five different dose levels
Cancer Res., 42, 5167–5171 (1982)

Sommer, H., Löffler, H.-P., Eisenbrand, G.
A method to determine N-nitrosoethanolamines in alkanolamines
J. Soc. Cosmet. Chem., 39, 133–137 (1988)

Spiegelhalder, B., Eisenbrand, G., Preussmann, R.
Contamination of amines with N-nitrosoamines
Angew. Chemie, 90, 379 (1978)
Int. Ed. (Engl.), 17, 367 (1978)

Sundlof, S.F., Mayhew, I.G.
A neuroparalytic syndrome associated with an oral flea repellant containing diethanolamine
Vet. Hum. Toxicol., 25, 247–249 (1983)

Story, D.L., Gee, S.J., Tyson, C.A., Gould, D.H.
Response of isolated hepatocytes to organic and inorganic cytotoxins
J. Toxicol. Environ. Health, 11, 483–501 (1983)

Windholz, M. (ed.)
The Merck Index, 10th ed., p. 451
Merck, Rahway (1983)

2-Methylpropene

1. Summary and assessment

2-Methylpropene is relatively quickly eliminated ($t_{0.5}$=1.3 hours, measured in the gas phase in a closed system). Accumulation occurs essentially in the brain and in the fat of the kidney glomerulus.

2-Methylpropene has a very low acute toxicity according to the reported studies o f inhalation in animals (LC_{50} in the mouse 178,000 ppm on 2 hours exposure; LC_{50} in the rat 266,000 ppm on 4 hours exposure). As a symptom of intoxication, states similar to narcosis can occur.

In a study of subacute oral toxicity in rats, no specific effects have been apparent at the highest tested dosage of 150 mg/kg.

In a sub-chronic inhalation study on rats, ketonuria has been detected at levels between 1,000 and 8,000 ppm. No specific effects have been found at the lowest test concentration of 250 ppm.

In point mutation assays in the Salmonella/microsome test, in *Escherichia coli* and in mouse lymphoma cells, there is no evidence of mutagenic activity.

Simultaneous exposure to 2-methylpropene and butane by inhalation leads to a synergistic effect (lethality) in animals.

In humans a retention of 17% has been found following inhalation of 100 ppm 2-methylpropene in the atmosphere.

2. Name of substance

2.1 Usual name	2-Methylpropene
2.2 IUPAC-name	2-Methylpropene
2.3 CAS-No.	115-11-7

3. Synonyms, common and trade names

isobutene
i-butylene
isobutylene
α-butylene
γ-butylene
asym-dimethyl ethylene

4.   Structural and molecular formulae

4.1   Structural formula

$$H_2C=\underset{\underset{\displaystyle CH_3}{|}}{C}-CH_3$$

4.2   Molecular formula C_4H_8

5.   Physical and chemical properties

5.1	Molecular mass, g/mol	56.11
5.2	Melting point, °C	−140.3
5.3	Boiling point, °C	−6.90
5.4	Vapour pressure, hPa	2570 (at 20 °C)
5.5	Density, g/cm^2	0.5879 (20 °C; as liquid at 25 °C)
5.6	Solubility in water	very sparingly soluble
5.7	Solubility in organic solvents	miscible in any proportion with alcohols, ether, hydrocarbons
5.8	Solubility in fat	No information available
5.9	pH-value	No information available
5.10	Conversion factor	1 ppm $\overset{\wedge}{=}$ 2.23 mg/m^3 1 mg/m^3 $\overset{\wedge}{=}$ 0.43 ppm (at 25 °C and 1013 hPa) (Obenaus et al., 1985)

6.   Uses

Versatile starting material in the production of synthetic rubbers, fuel additives, plastics, adhesives and sealing compounds; manufacture of tert-butanol (Obenaus et al., 1985).

7.   Experimental results

7.1   Toxicokinetics and metabolism

In the rat (Sprague-Dawley, 2 animals) the following clinical parameters, determined in a closed system, were obtained for 2-methylpropene:

Table 1

Half-life ($t_{0.5}$)	1.3 hours	(n=3 determinations)
$K_{elimination}$	0.53 hours^{-1}	(n=3 determinations)
Clearance	2.80 litres/kg/hour	(n=3 determinations)

In these investigations, measurements were made of the decrease in the isobutene concentration in the gaseous phase (Frank et al., 1980).

In a study on the distribution of 2-methylpropene in the tissues of rats following inhalation of 620 mg 2-methylpropene/litre for 4 hours (approx. 266,000 ppm, concentration corresponded with the LC_{50} value established in this study) the following values were obtained:

Table 2. Tissue concentrations (Shugaev, 1969)

Organ	2-methylpropene concentration (mg %)	95% confidence interval (mg %)
Brain	126.0	89.9–169.1
Liver	77.0	61.6– 93.1
Kidney	63.7	52.1– 75.2
Spleen	59.1	50.2– 68.1
Glomerular capsule fat	219.0	188.9–249.1

In the mouse, the following value was obtained following inhalation of 415mg 2-methylpropene/litre for 2 hours (approx. 178,000 ppm)

Organ	2-methylpropene concentration (mg %)	95% confidence interval (mg %)
Brain	264.1	197.7–330.5

In the cat, 2-methylpropene concentrations of 36 to 94 mg % were obtained in the different regions of the brain. Inhalation exposure led to the death of the two animals used (no further details on dosing or on the time of death; Shugaev, 1969).

According to the authors, there was a correlation in the above-mentioned studies between the narcotising effect and the 2-methylpropene concentration measured in the tissues (Shugaev, 1969).

7.2 Acute and subacute toxicity

The following LC_{50} values were obtained for the rat and the mouse after inhalation of 2-methylpropene:

Table 3. LC_{50} values

Animal species	Duration of exposure	LC_{50}	95% confidence interval
Mouse	2 hours	415 mg/litre (=178,000 ppm)	314–546 mg/litre (=135,000–234,000 ppm)
Rat	4 hours	620 mg/litre (=266,000 ppm)	550–700 mg/litre (=236,000–300,000 ppm)

This report gives no information on the number of animals used or on the symptoms of poisoning (Shugaev, 1969).

In a further inhalation study the following results were obtained in mice (von Öttingen, 1940):

Table 2

Concentration[a]	Symptoms
30%	No side effects
40%	After 7 to 9 minutes, excitation phase, followed by narcosis
50%	After 2 to 2.25 minutes, immediate narcosis
60–70%	After 50 to 60 seconds, immediate narcosis

[a] No indication of whether the percentages were by weight or by volume.

7.3   Skin and mucous membrane effects
No information available.

7.4   Sensitization
No information available.

7.5   Subchronic and chronic toxicity

In a 4-week experiment, 5 male and 5 female Charles-River rats each received by stomach tube a daily dose (7 times per week) of 0, 1.49, 14.86 or 148.55 mg/kg, as a 0 to 5% solution in maize oil. Treatment had no effect on mortality, overt toxicity, food consumption or body-weight gain. In the case of the female rats receiving the highest dose, there was a significant decrease in leucocytes, but the figures fell within the range for historical controls. The same applied to the slightly raised blood sugar values for both males and females given the highest dose. Dissection and histological examination yielded no treatment-related results (Essochem, 1986).

In an inhalation study, 10 male and 10 female Charles-River rats were each exposed to 0, 250, 1000 or 8000 ppm 2-methylpropene (v/v) for 6 hours/day on 5 days/week for a period of 13 weeks. The mean analytical values were 2 ± 0.9, 251 ± 7.4, 1006 ± 20.3 or 7995 ± 121.2 ppm. The appearance, behaviour, food consumption and body-weight gain of the exposed animals were not different from the controls. In the case of the haematological and biochemical parameters, there were similarly no changes that could be related to treatment. Both male and female rats in the 1000 ppm group and male rats in the 8000 ppm group showed a significant increase in ketone bodies in the urine after 13 weeks (semi-quantitative determination, $p<0.05$ and <0.01, respectively). Although such a result is normally linked with disturbances in protein and fat metabolism, its biological significance was described as "uncertain" by the authors. Dissection, organ weights, and histological examination (control and highest dosage level only) did not reveal any treatment-related results. It was concluded that 2-methylpropene concentrations of 250 to 8000 ppm resulted in no significant evidence of toxicity (Essochem, 1982).

7.6   Genotoxicity

7.6.1 In vitro

2-Methylpropene was tested for mutagenic properties in 2 independent studies on Salmonella typhimurium TA 98, TA 100, TA 1535, TA 1537 and TA 1538 and Escherichia coli

WP2 uvrA/pkM101. In the first study the level of purity of the 2-methylpropene used was 99%. There were no data on the level of purity in the second study. Both studies were conducted with and without metabolic activation. 2-Methylpropene concentrations of 250 to 10,000 ppm and 5 to 100% in the atmosphere were used. Whereas in the first study no cytotoxicity occurred, in the second study 2-methylpropene caused cytotoxic effects at atmospheric concentrations of 80% and above. In neither experiment was there any indication that 2-methylpropene was mutagenic (Schimizu et al., 1985; Essochem, 1981 a).

No evidence of mutagenic activity was obtained in experiments using L5178Y mouse lymphoma cells, with and with out metabolic activation. Atmospheric concentrations of 6.25 to 100% 2-methylpropene (with 5% CO_2) were used. Cytotoxic effects occurred above a concentration of 6.25% (Essochem, 1981 b).

In a cell transformation test, 2-methylpropene was tested on C38/10T1/2 Clone 8 cells (mouse embryo fibroblasts) with and without metabolic activation. Atmospheric concentrations of 25 to 100% 2-methylpropene were used. In this experiment no evidence of cell transformation was obtained for 2-methylpropene (Essochem, 1981 c).

7.6.2 In vivo
      No information available.

7.7   Carcinogenicity
      No information available.

7.8   Reproductive toxicity
      No information available.

7.9   Effects on the immune system
      No information available.

7.10   Neurotoxicity
      No information available.

7.11   Other effects
In combination experiments on mice using the method of Zipf, inhalation of 2-methylpropene and butane led to a statistically significant ($p < 0.05$) synergism in relation to lethality. This phenomenon was more notable in rats than in mice. In the case of the animals dying prematurely, there was a correlation between the concentrations of 2-methylpropene and butane measured in the

brain and the deaths occurring as a result of narcosis. This effect was more marked in mice than in rats. In both experimental series 12 animals were used (Shugaev, 1969).

8.   Experience in humans

In 7 test subjects, 20-minute inhalation of 100 ppm 2-methylpropene resulted in an average of 17% retention as determined from the concentrations in the inhaled and exhaled air (Wagner, 1974).

References

Essochem Europe Inc.
Isobutylene: Ames-test for mutagenic activity with *Salmonella typhimurium* TA 1535, TA 100, TA 1537, TA 1538 and TA 98 and *Escherichia coli* WP2uvrA(pkM101)
Unpublished report (1981a)

Essochem Europe Inc.
Isobutylene: Assessment of mutagenic potential in the mouse lymphoma mutation assay
Unpublished report (1981b)

Essochem Europe Inc.
Isobutylene: Induction of morphological transformation in C3H/10T1/2 Clone 8 Cells
Unpublished report (1981c)

Essochem Europe Inc.
Isobutylene: 4 Week oral (gavage) toxicity study in the rat
Unpublished report (1986)

Essochem Europe Inc.
Isobutylene: 13 Week inhalation toxicity study in the rat
Unpublished report (1982)

Frank, H., Hintze, T., Bimboes, D., Remmer, H.
Monitoring lipid peroxidation by breath analysis: Endogenous hydrocarbons and their metabolic elimination
Toxicol. Appl. Pharmacol., 56, 337–344 (1980)

Obenaus, F., Droste, W., Neumeister, J.
Butenes in: Ullmann's Encyclopedia of Industrial Chemistry
5th ed., Vol. A4, p. 483–494
VCH, Weinheim (1985)

Shimizu, H., Suzuki, Y., Takemura, N., Goto, S., Matsushita, H.
The result of microbial mutation test for forty-three industrial chemi-
cals
Jpn. J. Ind. Health, 27, 400–419 (1985)

Shugaev, B.B.
Concentrations of hydrocarbons in tissues as a measure of toxicity
Arch. Environ. Health, 18, 878–882 (1969)
see also:
Shugaev, B.B.
Russ, Pharmacol. Toxicol., 30, 54–55 (1967)
Shugaev, B.B.
Farmakologija i Toksikologija, 30, 102–105 (1967)
Farmakologija i Toksikologija, 31, 360–363 (1968)

Von Oettingen, W.R.
Toxicity and potential dangers of aliphatic and aromatic hydrocar-
bons
Publ. Health Bull. No. 255 (1940)
cited in: Patty's Industrial Hygiene and Toxicology
Ed.: G. D. Clayton and F. E. Clayton
3rd edition, Vol. 2B.
John Wiley, New York (1982)

Wagner, H.M.
Retention einiger Kohlenwasserstoffe bei der Inhalation
Schr. Reihe Vers. Wass.-Boden-Lufthyg., 41, 225–229 (1974)

2-Ethylhexanal

1. Summary and assessment

On the basis of acute toxicity studies on animals exposed orally, dermally or by inhalation, 2-ethylhexanal is moderately toxic (LD_{50}, rats oral, between 2,626 and 3,730 mg/kg body weight; rabbits dermal, 4,135 mg/kg body weight; rats inhalation LC_{50} >4,000 ppm ($\hat{=}$ > 21 mg/l)).

Repeated administration of 2-ethylhexanal in the diet of rats (about 2,000 mg/kg body weight, administration period 3 weeks) leads to moderate peroxisome proliferation in the liver, as well as hypolipidaemia and hepatomegaly. However, it has been suggested that these effects can arise only in rodents and not in humans or rhesus monkeys, or only to a very slight extent.

Depending on the concentration, 2-ethylhexanal can have an irritant effect on the skin and eyes of animals. Strongly irritant effects are observed on the skin after 4 or 20 hours.

2-Ethylhexanal has no point-mutagenic effect in the Salmonella/microsome test using four strains, with or without metabolic activation.

Experiments are presently being conducted for the Employment Accident Insurance Fund of the Chemical Industry (BG-Chemie) on acute and sub-acute inhalation toxicity, including testing for peroxisome-induction and sensory testing of respiratory tract irritation.

2. Name of substance

2.1	Usual name	2-Ethylhexanal
2.2	IUPAC-name	2-Ethylhexanal
2.3	CAS-No.	123-05-7

3. Synonyms, common and trade names

Butyl ethyl acetaldehyde
2-Ethylcaproaldehyde

α-Ethylcaproaldehyde
Ethylbutylacetaldehyde
Ethylhexaldehyde
2-Ethylhexaldehyde
Octyl aldehyde

4.   Structural and molecular formulae

4.1 Structural formula

$$H_3C-CH_2-CH_2-CH_2-\underset{\underset{CH_2-CH_3}{|}}{CH}-C\begin{smallmatrix}\nearrow O\\\searrow H\end{smallmatrix}$$

4.2 Molecular formula

$C_8H_{16}O$

5.   Physical and chemical properties

5.1	Molecular mass, g/mol	128.24
5.2	Melting point, °C	−85 (BASF, 1988 b)
5.3	Boiling point, °C	163.4 (Sax, 1979)
5.4	Vapour pressure, hPa	2 (at 20 °C; Sax, 1979) 7 (at 50 °C; BASF, 1988 b)
5.5	Density, g/cm^3	0.822 (at 20 °C; BASF, 1988 b)
5.6	Solubility in water	<0.02% (Falbe and Payer, 1975)
5.7	Solubility in organic solvents	No information available
5.8	Solubility in fat	No information available
5.9	pH-value	−
5.10	Conversion factor	1 ppm $\hat{=}$ 5.34 mg/m^3 1 mg/m^3 $\hat{=}$ 0.19 ppm (at 25 °C and 1013 hPa)

6.   Uses

Intermediate for manufacture of 2-ethylhexanol, 2-ethylhexanoic acid, 2-ethylhexylamine, heterocyclics, pharmaceuticals and perfumes (Falbe and Payer, 1975).

7.　Experimental results

7.1　Toxicokinetics and metabolism
No information available.

7.2　Acute and subacute toxicity
After a single oral dose, the LD_{50} for rats was between 2626 and 3730 mg/kg body weight. In mice the LD_{50} was 246 mg/kg body weight after intraperitoneal injection (see table 1).

Acute symptoms of toxicity in mice included reeling, dyspnoea, tonic-clonic spasms, lying on the side or stomach and a narcotic-like condition. Deaths were delayed. In rats, reeling, lying on the stomach, diarrhoea and a narcotic-like state were seen. Post-mortem examination at the end of the 14-day observation period revealed no macroscopic effects in rats or mice (BASF, 1964).

The dermal LD_{50} for rabbits (six animals/dose) after a 4-day occlusive application to the clipped dorsal skin was 4135 mg/kg body weight (95% confidence limits 2790–6121 mg/kg body weight). No details were given of symptoms of toxicity (Smyth et al., 1951).

Inhalation exposure of six rats to 4000 ppm ($\hat{=}$ 21 mg/l) for 4 hours led to one death (Smyth et al., 1951).

In an inhalation risk test, an atmosphere enriched or saturated with 2-ethylhexanal (at 20° C) caused no deaths in 12 rats exposed for 8 hours. Slight irritation of the mucous membranes occurred, as well as a questionable narcotic effect. No macroscopic effects were revealed at autopsy (BASF, 1964).

In two studies on the rat (F-344), five or seven males received 2% (v/w) 2-ethylhexanal in the food for 3 weeks (about 2000 mg/kg body weight at an assumed food intake of 100 g/kg body weight). In each case, 13 animals served as controls. 2-Ethylhexanal led to a significant ($p \leq 0.05$) decrease in serum cholesterol (36.2 ± 3.9 mg/100 ml; control 46.1 ± 4.8) and serum triglyceride levels (47.4 ± 8.1 mg/100 ml; control 114.8 ± 17.8), as well as significantly increased catalase activity (63 ± 3.9 U/mg protein; control 44 ± 2.7; $p \leq 0.01$) and carnitine acetyltransferase activity (10.0 ± 0.9 U/mg protein; control 2.7 ± 0.5; $p \leq 0.001$) in the liver. At the end of the study, the relative liver weight was significantly ($p \leq 0.001$) increased. In addition, the ratio of mitochondria to peroxisomes changed from 5 : 1 (control) to 5 : 3 (Moody and Reddy, 1978, 1982).

However, Cohen and Graso (1981) suggested, that these effects can arise only in rodents and not in humans rhesus monkeys, or only to a very slight extent.

Table 1. Acute toxicity of 2-ethylhexanal

Species	Number of animals/ dose	Sex	Route of exposure	Observation period	LD$_{50}$	References
Mouse	–	♂, ♀	intra- peritoneal	14 days	0.3 ml/kg body weight ($\hat{=}$ 246 mg/kg body weight)	BASF, 1964
Rat	–	♂, ♀	oral	14 days	3.2 ml/kg body weight ($\hat{=}$ 2626 mg/kg body weight)	BASF, 1964
Rat	5	–	oral	14 days	3730 mg/kg body weight (95% confidence limits: 2430–5740 mg/kg body weight)	Smyth et al., 1951
Rabbit	6	–	dermal	14 days	5.04 ml/kg body weight ($\hat{=}$ 4135 mg/kg body weight 95% confidence limits: 2790–6121 mg/kg body weight)	Smyth et al., 1951

– no details available

7.3   Skin and mucous membrane effects

Neat 2-ethylhexanal led to marked reddening of the skin of rabbits after a 1-, 5- or 15-minute dorsal application, with spreading oedema formation (seen after 24 hours). Eight days after exposure, marked flaking of the skin was still present. A 20-hour exposure (semi-occlusive) led to focal necroses. The area surrounding the application site showed marked reddening and oedema formation. Eight days after treatment, the damaged skin was still not completely healed (BASF, 1964).

In a further study on rabbits (two females) a test patch (ca 2 cm^2) loaded with 500 µl 2-ethylhexanal was applied to the clipped dorsal skin. At the end of the 4-hour semi-occlusive application, marked reddening and oedema formation were seen in the test animals. These effects remained almost unchanged for the first two days of the observation period, but cleared in the course of a week. No necrosis was seen. There were no systemic signs of toxicity due to absorption (BASF, 1978).

A 24-hour occlusive application of 500 µl undiluted 2-ethyl-hexanal to the clipped dorsal skin of five rabbits (five animals) resulted in marked erythema, oedema formation and necrosis (Smyth et al., 1951).

More recent studies on the irritant effects of neat 2-ethylhexanal in the rabbit (OECD-method 404) produced reddening, oedema and crust formation (irritation index 6.08 out of a maximum of 8) after a 4-hour application. The substance was judged to be a severe irritant (Hüls, 1986).

Instillation of 50 µl of neat 2-ethylhexanal into the conjunctival sac of rabbits led to slight reddening of the eye and oedema formation after one hour. Twenty-four hours after instillation, marked reddening was observed, which completely disappeared after 8 days (BASF, 1964).

In a further investigation in rabbit's eyes, slight irritation (no further details) was seen 24 hours after instillation of 500 µl undiluted 2-ethylhexanal into the conjunctival sac (Smyth et al., 1951).

In more recent investigations of eye irritation (OECD method 405), 2-ethylhexanal caused slight reddening and swelling of the conjunctiva, slight clouding of the cornea and slight iritis (irritation index 13.58 out of a maximum of 110). The product was judged to be slightly irritating (Hüls, 1986).

7.4   Sensitization
No information available.

7.5   Subchronic and chronic toxicity
No information available.

7.6   Genotoxicity

7.6.1 In vitro
2-Ethylhexanal (purity not specified) was tested for point-mutagenic activity in the Salmonella/microsome test in strains TA 97, TA 98, TA 100 and TA 1535 using a pre-incubation protocol, both with and without metabolic activation. Doses employed were 0 (control), 3000, 10,000, 33,000, 100,000, 166,000, 333,000, and 666,000 µg/plate. S9 mix from Aroclor-induced Sprague-Dawley rat or Syrian hamster livers served as the metabolizing system. In each case, the S9 mix contained either 10% or 30% S9. 2-Ethylhexanal is not point-mutagenic under these conditions (Zeiger et al., 1988).

7.6.2 In vivo
No information available.

7.7   Carcinogenicity
No information available.

7.8   Reproductive toxicity
No information available.

7.9   Effects on the immune system
No information available.

7.10   Neurotoxicity
No information available.

7.11   Other effects
No information available.

8.   Experience in humans

According to one manufacturer, there is no information of sensitization by 2-ethylhexanal, either in the factory or in the company medical department (BASF, 1988 a).

References

BASF AG
Toxicology Department
Unpublished studies (1964)

BASF AG
Toxicology Department
Unpublished studies (1978)

BASF AG
Communication from the Department of Occupational Medicine &
Health Protection (1988 a)

BASF AG
Safety data sheet "2-Ethylhexanal" (1988 b)

Cohen, A.J., Grasso, P.
Review of the hepatic response to hypolipidaemic drugs in rodents
and assessment of its toxicological significance to man
Food Cosmet. Toxicol., 19, 585–605 (1981)

Falbe, J., Payer, W.
Aldehyde, aliphatische
in: Ullmann's Enzyklopedie der technischen Chemie
4th edition, volume 7, p. 130 (1975)
Verlag Chemie, Weinheim

Hüls AG
Unpublished reports (1986)

Moody, D.E., Reddy, J.K.
Hepatic peroxisome (microbody) proliferation in rats fed plasticizers
and related compounds
Toxicol. Appl. Pharmacol., 45, 497–504 (1978)

Moody, D.E., Reddy, J.K.
Serum triglyceride and cholesterol contents in male rats receiving
diets containing plasticizers and analogues of the ester 2-ethylhexa-
nol
Toxicol. Lett., 10, 379–383 (1982)

Sax, N.I. (ed.)
Dangerous Properties of Industrial Materials
5th edition
van Nostrand Reinhold Company (1979)

Smyth, H.F., Carpenter, C.P., Weil, C.S.
Range-finding toxicity data: List IV
Arch. Ind. Health, 4, 119–122 (1951)

Zeiger, E., Anderson, B., Haworth, S., Lawlor, T., Mortelmans, K.
Salmonella mutagenicity tests: IV. Results from the testing of 300 chemicals
Environ. Molecul. Mutagen., 11, Suppl. 12, 1–158 (1988)

Maleic acid dimethyl ester

1. Summary and assessment

Following acute oral and dermal application the substance proves to be of low systemic toxicity (oral LD_{50} 1410 mg/kg (rat), 1340 mg/kg (mouse), dermal LD_{50} 530 mg/kg (rabbit) and >2000 mg/kg (rat)).

In two skin-irritation tests with somewhat differing results the substance is at most slightly irritant following a single application and shows a sensitising potential on guinea pigs.

Following repeated dermal treatment (20 applications), a leucocytosis is manifested systemically in the rat, as well as depletion of glutathione-SH in liver cells. Dependent on the dose, erythema and oedema occur locally followed by necrosis. Histopathological findings include dermatitis, acanthosis and also hyperkeratosis.

In in vitro investigations on various bacterial strains, both with and without metabolic activation, the substance shows no point-mutagenic effect. In the micronucleus test on the mouse it causes no chromosomal aberrations.

2. Name of substance

2.1	Usual name	Maleic acid dimethyl ester
2.2	IUPAC-name	Z-Ethene dicarboxylic acid dimethyl ester
2.3	CAS-No.	624-48-6

3. Synonyms, common and trade names

But(2)ene-1,4-dicarboxylic acid dimethyl ester
Dimethylmaleinat
Dimethyl maleate
Methyl maleate
Sipomer
DMM
MAD

4. Structural and molecular formulae

4.1 Structural formula

$$
\begin{array}{c}
\quad\quad\;\; O \\
\quad\quad\;\; \| \\
HC\!-\!C\!-\!OCH_3 \\
\; | \\
HC\!-\!C\!-\!OCH_3 \\
\quad\quad\;\; \| \\
\quad\quad\;\; O
\end{array}
$$

4.2 Molecular formula

$C_6H_8O_4$

5. Physical and chemical properties

5.1	Molcecular mass	114.14 g/mol
5.2	Melting point, °C	−19
5.3	Boiling point, °C	202
5.4	Vapour pressure, hPa	1.33 (at 45.7 °C)
5.5	Density, g/cm³	1.1606 (at 20 °C)
5.6	Solubility in water	insoluble, hydrolysed slowly
5.7	Solubility in organic solvents	soluble in ether
5.8	Solubility in fat	readily soluble
5.9	pH-value	–
5.10	Conversion factor	$1\ mg/m^3 \;\hat{=}\; 0.17\ ppm$
		$1\ ppm \;\hat{=}\; 5.89\ mg/m^3$
		(at 25 °C and 1013 hPa)
		(Weast, 1981/82; Sax, 1979)

6. Uses

Intermediate product for the manufacture of dispersants, succinic acid dimethyl ester and acetyl succinic acid dimethyl ester
(Hoechst, 1981).

7. Experimental results

7.1 Toxicokinetics and metabolism
No information available.

7.2   Acute and subacute toxicity

The acute oral LD_{50} in the male rat (Carworth-Wistar) was 1410 mg/kg for a 14-day period of observation (Smyth et al., 1962). For male and female mice the oral LD_{50} of maleic acid dimethyl ester was established as 1340 mg/kg. Death occurred within 4 days of application. Symptoms occurring during LD_{50} determination were: reduced spontaneous activity, apathy, ventral position and ptosis, and in some animals shortness of breath and a ruffled coat (LMP, 1982).

In the case of the rabbit the dermal LD_{50} following 24-hour skin contact (substance beneath a plastic film) and a 14-day period of observation was given as 530 mg/kg (Smyth et al., 1962).

For rats a LD_{50} of >2000 mg/kg was obtained under occlusive conditions (RCC, 1985 a).

5 Male and female rats per group (Wistar, 9 to 11 weeks old, body weight 216 to 238 g and 183 to 215 g, respectively) were shaved on the back prior to application. A volume of 2 ml/kg body weight of maleic acid dimethyl ester in olive oil was applied to the skin daily for 6 hours on 5 days/week (total 20 applications) in the following doses: 0 (vehicle control), 60, 170 and 500 mg/kg. The area of application amounted to approximately 10% of the body surface and was covered occlusively following application. The programme of investigation corresponds with OECD Guideline 410 of 12. 5. 1981. No treatment-related deaths or systemic symptoms were observed. Dose-dependent local effects ranged from slight erythema and desquamation in the lowest dose groups to well-marked erythema, slight to moderate oedema and desquamation and slight to well-marked necrosis in the highest dose group. The male rats in the middle and highest dose groups showed a significant decrease in food consumption and body-weight gain, an effect which was not observed in the females. The haematological results obtained gave indications of slight leucocytosis (increase in the white blood cells accompanied by a slight increase in the neutrophil leucocytes and a decrease in lymphocytes in the differential blood picture) in animals in the highest dose group. The biochemical investigation showed the chief effect to be a moderate depletion of oxidised hepatic glutathione (GSSH) and a correlated decrease in the total hepatic glutathione (GSH+GSSH) in the highest dose group. Further blood anomalies (thromboplastin, partial thromboplastin time, electrolytes, glucose, urea, transferase) were observed in this group, but these were interpreted by the author as secondary effects. Urine analysis

yielded no treatment-related anomalies. Absolute and relative organ weights differed in some cases, but no clear target organ could be identified in relation to the above-mentioned effects. The microscopic studies showed no treatment-related effects except for the skin changes in the middle and highest dose groups. Associated with the macroscopic results obtained, some animals in the middle dose group showed slight dermatitis, acanthosis and hyperkeratosis, while all animals in the highest dose group showed moderate dermatitis and moderately well- to clearly-marked necroses. Although the systemic "no effect level" was established as 60 mg/kg body weight, the actual level must be less than this when the local effects on the skin are taken into account (RCC, 1987).

In further investigations in rats (Hoechst, 1984, no further details), maleic acid dimethyl ester caused inflammatory reddening of the skin following dermal application and corrosion and bleeding of the gastrointestinal tract following oral administration of high doses (1400 mg/kg).

7.3   Skin and mucous membrane effects

In investigations on the irritant effect on the rabbit (BASF, 1982, no further details) the substance caused slight skin and mucosal irritation. The skin irritation test conducted according to OECD Guideline No. 404 (RCC, 1985 b) resulted in transient slight erythema or oedema formation in the rabbit (evaluation after 1 hour).

Maleic acid dimethyl ester caused slight irritation (graded 3 on a 10-point scale) on application to the cornea of the rabbit eye (0.1–0.5 ml, examination of the eye after 24 hours; Carpenter and Smyth, 1946).

7.4   Sensitization

15 Female guinea pigs (Pirbright-White, body weight 276–328 g) were used in the maximisation test (treatment group: 10; control group: 5). A concentration of 1% maleic acid dimethyl ester (used for the intradermal and dermal induction as well as dermal challenge) caused 48 and 72 hours after challenge very slight to severe erythema including escher formation and edema. Maleic has to be regarded therefore as a potential skin sensitizer (Hoechst, 1989).

7.5   Subchronic and chronic toxicity

No information available.

7.6   Genotoxicity

7.6.1 In vitro

In the Salmonella/microsome test, maleic acid dimethyl ester was not found to be mutagenic in strains TA 1537, TA 1538, TA 98, TA 1535 and TA 100, either with or without the addition of S9-Mix from Aroclor-induced rat liver. The concentrations tested were 50, 250, 1250 and 5000 µg/plate (LMP, 1982a).

7.6.2 In vivo

In the micronucleus test on male and female NMRI mice (10 animals/group) maleic acid dimethyl ester showed no genotoxic effect. Micronucleus formation was determined in polychromatic erythrocytes from the bone marrow 24, 48 and 72 hours after oral administration of 1000 mg maleic acid diemthyl ester/kg (=0.75 LD_{50}). A toxic effect on the bone marrow (decrease in polychromatic erythrocytes) and also symptoms consistent with acute toxicity (apathy, ventral position, ptosis, ruffled coat, shortness of breath) were observed in these experiments (LMP, 1982b).

7.7   Carcinogenicity
No information available.

7.8   Reproductive toxicity
No information available.

7.9   Effects on the immune system
No information available.

7.10 Neurotoxicity
No information available.

7.11 Other effects
No information available.

8.   Experience in humans

No information available.

References

BASF AG
Communication to BG Chemie
Dated 19. 1. 1982

Carpenter, C.P., Smyth, H.F.
Chemical burns of the rabbit cornea
Am. J. Ophthalmol., 29, 1363 (1946)

Hoechst AG
Safety data sheet, April 1981

Hoechst AG
Communication to BG Chemie
Dated 5. 7. 1984

Hoechst AG
Maleinsäuredimethylester – Prüfung auf sensibilisierende Eigen-
schaften an Pirbright-White-Meerschweinchen im Maximierungstest
Unveröffentlichter Bericht Nr. 89.1710 (1989)
Commissioned by BG Chemie

LMP (Laboratory for Mutagenicity Testing, Darmstadt Technical
University)
Testing the substance maleic acid dimethyl ester for mutagenicity in
the Ames test and micronucleus test
commissioned by BG Chemie
Report of 12. 11. 1982a, b

RCC (Research and Consultant Company, Itingen)
Maleic acid dimethylester – Acute dermal toxicity study in rats
Project 035910 (1985 a)
Commissioned by BG Chemie

RCC (Research and Consultant Company, Itingen)
Maleic acid dimethylester – Primary skin irritation study in rabbits
Project 045696 (1985 b)
Commissioned by BG Chemie

RCC (Research and Consultant Company, Itingen)
Maleic acid dimethylester – Subacute 28 days repeated dermal
toxicity in rats
Project 035897 (1987)
Commissioned by BG Chemie

Sax, N.I. (ed.)
Dangerous properties of industrial materials
Van Nostrand Reinhold, New York (1979)

Smyth, H.F., Carpenter, C.P., Weil, C.S., Pozzani, U.C., Striese, J.A.
Range-Finding toxicity data: list VI
Am. Ind. Hyg. Assoc. J., 23, 95 (1962)

Weast, R.C. (ed.)
CRC-Handbook of Chemistry and Physics, 62nd ed., C-364
CRC, Boca Raton, Florida (1981/82)

Trimethylquinone

1. Summary and assessment

The acute oral LD_{50} of trimethylquinone in the rat is approximately 300 mg/kg body weight, the animals developing dyspnoe and dizziness. On subsequent examination, caustic damage to the stomach wall and adhesions between the stomach and surrounding organs are observed. A single intraperitoneal injection results in an LD_{50} of approximately 18 mg/kg body weight in the mouse, with dyspnoea and cramps and, on subsequent examination, adhesions in the abdominal cavity. After a single dermal application of trimethylquinone in the rabbit, an LD_{50} of <200 mg/kg body weight is obtained, the caustic action producing local necroses. Other effects include accelerated breathing, cyanosis of the extremities and apathy. On dissection, lung oedema, acute dilation with congestive hyperaemia of the heart and petechial haemorrhages in the thymus are observed. In rats, the inhalation of an atmosphere trimethylquinone vapour saturated at 100° C does not result in mortality after 1 hour of exposure, but after 3 and 8 hours the number of deaths are 1/6 and 4/6 animals, respectively. The exposed animals suffer irritation of the mucous membranes and shortness of breath, and they show evasive behaviour. Inhalation exposure to an atmosphere saturated or enriched at 20° C is tolerated for 8 hours, the only effect noted being irritation of the eyes.

Trimethylquinone is highly caustic to the skin and eyes of rabbits.

In the guinea-pig, trimethylquinone has demonstrated sensitising potential.

In the Ames test, both with and without metabolic activation (S9 mix), trimethylquinone does not induce point-mutations at concentrations of up to 5000 µg/plate in the standard plate test or 500 µg/plate in the pre-incubation test. A bacteriotoxic effect is observed in the standard plate test at 500 µg/plate, and in the pre-incubation test at 100–250 µg/plate (without S9 mix), or at 500 µg/plate (with S9 mix).

In human lymphocytes, abnormal chromosome configurations and polyploidy are observed after in vitro exposure to trimethylquinone, indicating genotoxic activity.

In isolated rat liver mitochondria, trimethylquinone causes the depletion of calcium ions and of glutathione, with subsequent swelling of the mitochondria. The authors conclude from the results that the substance is toxic to the hepatocytes.

Skin changes have been observed in man after occupational exposure to trimethylquinone.

The principal toxic effect of trimethylquinone is its caustic action on the skin and eyes. Trimethylquinone is a skin sensitiser, and is absorbed by the skin. It is toxic after oral and dermal absorption. Vapours produced at 100 °C cause fatalities in the rat, with local damage to the respiratory tract. There are indications that trimethylquinone is clastogenic. In man, skin irritation has been observed as a result of handling the chemical.

2.   Name of substance

2.1 Usual name	Trimethylquinone
2.2 IUPAC-name	2,3,5-Trimethylcyclohexa-2,5-diene-1,4-dione
2.3 CAS-No.	935-92-2

3.   Synonyms, common and trade names

p-Pseudocumoquinone
Trimethylbenzoquinone
Trimethylchinon
2,3,6-Trimethylquinone
2,3,5-Trimethyl-2,5-cyclohex-adiene-1,4-dione
2,3,5-Trimethyl-p-benzoquin-one

4.   Structural and molecular formulae

4.1 Structural formula

4.2 Molecular formula $C_9H_{10}O_2$

5.   Physical and chemical properties

5.1	Molecular mass, g/mol	116.16
5.2	Melting point, °C	32 (BASF, 1987)
5.3	Boiling point, °C	100 (at 20 hPa) (BASF, 1987)
5.4	Vapour pressure, hPa	2.5 (at 20 °C) (BASF, 1987)
5.5	Density, g/cm^3	1.08 (at 20 °C) (BASF, 1987)
5.6	Solubility in water	low (BASF, 1987)
5.7	Solubility in organic solvents	soluble in acetone (BASF, 1970)
5.8	Solubility in fat	No information available
5.9	pH-value	No information available
5.10	Conversion factor	1 ppm $\hat{=}$ 4.82 mg/m^3 1 mg/m^3 $\hat{=}$ 0.21 ppm (at 25 °C and 1013 hPa)

6.   Uses

Starting material in the synthesis of trimethyl hydroquinone for manufacturing synthetic Vitamin E preparations (Ernst et al., 1983).

7.   Experimental results

7.1   Toxicokinetics and metabolism
No information available.

7.2   Acute and subacute toxicity
The acute oral toxicity of trimethylquinone was investigated in the rat (no data on strain, sex or number of animals), providing an LD_{50} value of approx. 300 mg/kg body weight. Dyspnoea and reeling were observed as symptoms of toxicity. Autopsy revealed caustic damage to the stomach wall and adhesions between the stomach and surrounding organs (BASF, 1969).

In the mouse, an intraperitoneal LD_{50} value of approx. 18 mg/kg body weight was obtained (no data on strain, sex or number of animals). The main toxic symptoms were dyspnoea and violent cramps. Intra-abdominal adhesions were among the findings at autopsy (BASF, 1969).

A dose of 200 mg trimethylquinone/kg body weight (as a 50% aqueous preparation) was applied to the intact skin of five male and five female rabbits. The animals were clipped the previous day, and the material was applied to the back and shoulders, covering an area of 50 cm^2. Within 24 hours, skin necrosis was evident, and all the animals developed accelerated breathing, cyanosis of the ears, nose and snout, and apathy. They all died within 24 hours. Subsequent examination revealed slight oedema of the lungs, acute dilation of the heart with congestive hyperaemia, and petechial haemorrhages in the thymus. The heart and lungs were bronze coloured. The median lethal dose (LD$_{50}$) after dermal application was therefore <200 mg/kg body weight (BASF, 1978).

The acute inhalation toxicity of trimethylquinone was assessed in rats (no data on strain and sex) exposed for 1, 3 or 8 hours to an atmosphere saturated at 20° C and at 100° C with the volatile components of trimethylquinone. For saturation purposes, air was passed through a 5 cm-deep layer of trimethylquinone at a rate of 200 l/hour. The trimethylquinone/air mixture saturated at 20° C caused slight eye irritation after 8 hours of exposure (no data are available on the observation period). All of the 12 rats survived. Subsequent examination did not reveal any pathological changes. The trimethylquinone/air mixture saturated at 100° C did not result in any deaths after 1 hour of exposure, but 1/6 and 4/6 rats died after 3 and 8 hours of exposure, respectively. Toxicity was characterised by severe irritation of the mucous membranes, shortness of breath and evasive behaviour. On dissection, the animals that died prematurely had soiled snouts and front paws and dilated gastro-intestinal tracts, whilst the other animals displayed no macroscopically-visible effects (BASF, 1969).

7.3   Skin and mucous membrane effects

The skin compatibility of trimethylquinone was tested on the clipped dorsal skin of white rabbits, in the rag test. A cotton cloth (2.5 cm^2) soaked in neat trimethylquinone (melted in a water bath) was applied once for 1, 5, or 15 minutes or for 20 hours to the skin of four rabbits (no further data). Twenty-four hours after exposure for 1, 5 or 15 minutes, the application site showed slight reddening, marked oedema formation and haemorrhaging. After 8 days, irrespective of the duration of the application, slight to marked necroses had formed, which displayed a blister-like appearance. Application for 20 hours resulted in severe oedema formation and the deaths of three out of the four rabbits, within 24 hours (no further data). After 8 days, prominent necrosis of the dorsal skin was evident. When the ears of rabbits were treated in the same way (20-hour application), marked discoloration was seen after 24 hours and marked necrosis after 8 days (BASF, 1969).

The irritant effect of trimethylquinone on the mucous membranes was tested by melting the substance and instilling 50 µl of the neat liquid into the conjunctival sac of one eye of the rabbit. Physiological saline was instilled into the other eye for comparison (no data on the number of animals). Whilst no irritation was evident in the control eye, severe oedema of the experimental eye developed within one hour, so that the eyeball could no longer be distinguished. After 24 hours, marked redness, haemorrhages, and marked corneal opacity had developed in addition to the severe oedema, with only a marginal improvement after 8 days (BASF, 1969).

7.4 Sensitization

A sensitization test was conducted in 13 female guinea-pigs (ten test animals and three controls) that were shaved over an area of approx. 25 cm^2 on the right and left upper flanks. After a single application to the left flank of a 10% solution of trimethylquinone in acetone, the same area was subsequently brushed eight times in 4 days with a 1% solution (again, in acetone). This resulted in the development of bloody scabs. After 12 days, the previously un-treated right flank was brushed with a 0.1% solution. No reactions were seen. After a further 5 days the right flank was treated with a 1% solution (primarily non-irritating), and all ten guinea-pigs developed a clear reddening of the skin, with slight swelling around the application site, indicating a sensitization reaction to trimethylquinone (BASF, 1970).

7.5   Subchronic and chronic toxicity
No information available.

7.6   Genotoxicity

7.6.1 In vitro

2,3,6-Trimethylquinone (purity 99%) was tested for point-mutagenic activity in the Ames test on *Salmonella typhimurium* in strains TA 98, TA 100, TA 1535 and TA 1537. Five concentrations were tested in the standard plate test: from 20 to 5000 µg/plate in strains TA 98 and TA 100, both with and without metabolic activation by S9 mix (containing microsomal enzymes from Aroclor 1254-induced rat livers); from 0.8 to 500 µg/plate in strains TA 98, TA 100, TA 1535 and TA 1537, without metabolic activation; from 4 to 1500 µg/plate in strains TA 98, TA 100, TA 1535 and TA 1537 with metabolic activation. In a pre-incubation test in strains TA 98, TA 100, TA 1535 and TA 1537 concentrations of 0.8 to 250 µg/plate were tested without metabolic activation, and 4 to 500 µg/plate with metabolic activation by S9 mix. In all the experiments, DMSO was used as the solvent. Trimethylquinone was bacteriotoxic in the standard plate test (after 48 hours of incubation at 37° C) from 500 µg/plate, and in the pre-incubation test from 100 to 250 µg/plate without S9 mix and from 500 µg/plate with S9 mix. No point-mutagenic activity was seen in any of the experiments described (BASF, 1989).

The clastogenic effect of 10 µg trimethylquinone/ml of medium was tested on human lymphocytes from 72-hour-old cultures after 6 hours of incubation, or after 60 or 90 minutes of intermittent exposure, followed by a recovery period of 8 and 24 hours respectively. After intermittent exposure for 90 minutes with a 24-hour recovery phase, varying quadriradial chromosome configurations were observed, with polyploidies in the metaphase (Drets et al., 1982).

7.6.2 In vivo
No information available.

7.7   Carcinogenicity
No information available.

7.8   Reproductive toxicity
No information available.

7.9   Effects on the immune system
No information available.

7.10   Neurotoxicity
No information available.

7.11 Other effects
On isolated liver mitochondria of male Sprague-Dawley rats, a 500 µM trimethylquinone solution ($\hat{=}$ 58.1 µg/ml of DMSO plus water) gave rise to extensive glutathione depletion and calcium ion draining, followed by mitochondrial swelling, which the authors attributed to a cytotoxic activity of trimethylquinone on the hepatocytes (Moore et al., 1987).

8.   Experience in humans

Skin aberrations have been observed in workers handling trimethylquinone (no further data; BASF, 1970).

9.   Threshold limit values

No information available.

References

BASF AG, Toxicology Department
Ergebnis der gewerbetoxikologischen Vorprüfung (XIX/9)
Unpublished study (1969)

BASF AG, Toxicology Department
Bericht über die Prüfung von Trimethylchinon und Trimethylhydro-
chinon auf hautsensibilisierende Wirkung (XIX/9–10)
Unpublished study (1970)

BASF AG, Toxicology Department
Bericht über die Prüfung der akuten dermalen Toxizität von Trime-
thylchinon an der Rückenhaut weißer Kaninchen (77/748)
Unpublished study (1978)

BASF AG
Trimethylchinon
Grunddatensatz für Großstoffe, dated 2. 10. 1987

BASF AG, Toxicology Department
Report on the study of 2,3,6-trimethylquinone in the Ames test
(standard plate test and preincubation test with *Salmonella typhimu-
rium*)
Project No.: 40110727/884315
Unpublished study (1989)

Drets, M.E., Folle, G.A., Aznarez, A.
Clastogenic action of a dimethyl p-benzoquinone of animal origin
Mutat. Res., 102, 159–172 (1982)

Ernst, H.G., Florent, J., Fürst, A., Häfner, H., Kuhn, W. Meier, W.,
Paust, J., Pollak, P., Reiff, F., Suter, C.
Vitamine
Ullmanns Enzyklopädie der technischen Chemie
Vol. 23, p. 646
Verlag Chemie, Weinheim (1983)

Moore, G.A., Rossi, L., Nicotera, P., Orrenius, S., O'Brien, P.J.
Quinone toxicity in hepatocytes: studies on mitochondrial Ca^{2+} release induced by benzoquinone derivatives
Arch. Biochem. Biophys., 259, 283–295 (1987)

2,4-Dinitromethylaniline

1. Summary and assessment

2,4-Dinitromethylaniline is of low acute toxicity on oral administration (LD_{50} rat, oral, 1330 or 2000 mg/kg). The symptoms following acute administration indicate an effect on the central nervous system.

The chemical shows no irritation activity on the skin or mucous membranes.

2,4-Dinitromethylaniline induces point mutations in the Ames test with and without metabolic activation, but is not mutagenic to E. coli. A chromosomal aberration test with Chinese hamster V 79 cells is negative.

Acute dermal administration to cats does not induce methaemoglobin-formation, but does produce anaemia (reduced haemoglobin level and numbers of erythrocytes, increased numbers of reticulocytes and Heinz bodies).

2. Name of substance

2.1 Usual name   2,4-Dinitromethylaniline

2.2 IUPAC-name   N-Methyl-2,4-dinitroaniline

2.3 CAS-No.   2044-88-4

3. Synonyms, common and trade names

2,4-Dinitro-1-methyl-amino-benzene
N-Methyl-2,4-dinitrobenzen-amine
2,4-Dinitro-N-methylaniline

4.   Structural and molecular formulae

4.1 Structural formula

$$HN-CH_3$$

(benzene ring with substituents: NO_2 at position 2, NO_2 at position 4)

4.2 Molecular formula $C_7H_7N_3O_4$

5.   Physical and chemical properties

5.1 Molecular mass, g/mol	197
5.2 Melting point, °C	175 (Beilstein, 1929)
5.3 Boiling point, °C	No information available
5.4 Vapour pressure, hPa	No information available
5.5 Density, g/cm^3	No information available
5.6 Solubility in water	Slightly soluble in hot water (Beilstein, 1929)
5.7 Solubility in organic solvents	Soluble in acetone, alcohol and methanol hardly soluble in benzene (Beilstein, 1950)
5.8 Solubility in fat	No information available
5.9 pH-value	ca. 7 in aqueous solution (Hoechst, 1982)
5.10 Conversion factor	$1\ mg/m^3 \mathrel{\hat{=}} 0.12\ ppm$ $1\ ppm \mathrel{\hat{=}} 8.06\ mg/m^3$ (at 25 °C and 1013 hPa)

6.   Uses

Intermediate used in manufacture of explosives (Hoechst, 1982).

7.   Experimental results

7.1 Toxicokinetics and metabolism
No information available.

7.2   Acute and subacute toxicity

The acute oral LD_{50} for 2,4-dinitromethylaniline has been determined in Wistar rats as >2000 mg/kg body weight in males and 1330 mg/kg body weight in females. Clinical symptoms included reduced spontaneous activity, ruffled fur, crouching posture, drawn in flanks, uncoordinated and reeling movement, cringing behaviour, irregular breathing, eye irritation, lying on the stomach or side, and confusion. In addition, the frequency of breathing was reduced. Encrustation of the edges of the eyelids and the nostrils was seen, as well as trembling and tonic-clonic spasms. Death occurred up to 9 days after administration. The females were affected more than the males (Hoechst, 1988 c).

7.3   Skin and mucous membrane effects

Three albino New Zealand rabbits (weight 2.3–3.1 kg, 3–5 months old, sex not given) received 500 mg 2,4-dinitromethylaniline made into a paste with 0.3 ml of a 0.9% sodium chloride solution. This was applied semi-occlusively to the shaved back for 4 hours. The skin reaction was assessed 30–60 minutes after removal of the plaster and at 24, 48 and 72 hours. One hour after removal of the plaster, the treated skin was very slightly reddened and stained light yellow. There were no signs of irritation 24 hours after removal of the plaster (Hoechst, 1988 a).

Three albino New Zealand rabbits (weight 2.8–3.6 kg, 3–5 months old, sex not given) each had 100 mg 2,4-dinitromethylaniline instilled into the conjunctival sac of the left eye. The untreated eye served as a control. Evaluation of the eyes took place at 1, 24, 48 and 72 hours after application. After 24 and 72 hours, the cornea was examined for damage under UV light after instillation of a drop of fluorescein sodium solution. Effects on the conjunctiva ranged from acute slight swelling and a clear hyperaemia of the blood vessels, to a crimson red colouration of the entire conjunctiva. The irises of all the animals were reddened. The conjunctiva of all the animals were clearly congested 24 hours after instillation, and that of one animal 48 hours after instillation. All symptoms of irritation were reversed 72 hours after instillation (Hoechst, 1988 b).

7.4   Sensitization

No information available.

7.5   Subchronic and chronic toxicity

No information available.

7.6   Genotoxicity

7.6.1 In vitro

2,4-Dinitromethylaniline was tested for point-mutagenic activity in the *Salmonella typhimurium* strains TA 100, TA 1535, TA 1537, TA 1538 and TA 98 and in *Escherichia coli* WP2uvrA. The mutagenicity study was carried out with and without activation by microsomal fractions from rat liver homogenates. Concentrations of 0.16, 0.8, 4, 20, 100 and 500 µg/plate were used. Bacteriotoxicity was evident at concentrations of 500 µg/plate and above. The results showed that the chemical caused a dose-dependent point-mutagenic effect in all strains both with and without metabolic activation. Investigations on *Escherichia coli* showed no comparable effect (Hoechst, 1988 e).

In an in vitro chromosomal aberration assay on V79 cells of the Chinese hamster, 2,4-dinitromethylaniline was tested with and without metabolic activation. The following doses were used: without metabolic activation 6, 12.5 and 25 µg/ml; with metabolic activation 250, 500 and 1000 µg/ml. The results showed that the substance did not induce any significant increase in the number of chromosome aberrations, whether or not a metabolic activation system was added (Hoechst, 1988 d).

7.6.2 In vivo
No information available.

7.7   Carcinogenicity
No information available.

7.8   Reproductive toxicity
No information available.

7.9   Effects on the immune system
No information available.

7.10   Neurotoxicity
No information available.

7.11   Other effects

Doses of 50 or 200 mg 2,4-dinitromethylaniline/kg body weight were administered orally to groups of two female cats (SPF strain, no further details). Blood was removed from the ear vein immediately before administration and at 10 and 30 minutes, 1, 3 and 5 hours and 1, 2, 3, 4, 7 and 14 days after administration. The following parameters were assessed: erythrocyte count, haemoglobin content, haematocrit level, average haemoglobin content of the erythrocytes, average erythrocyte volume and concentration, average haemoglobin concentration, leukocyte count, platelet count, reticulocyte count, Heinz bodies and methaemoglobin level. In addition to this, a differential blood cell count was made. Neither dose of 2,4-dinitromethylaniline produced any measurable formation of methaemoglobin. In the animals treated with 50 mg/kg body weight, there were no substance-related haematological changes observed. One of the cats given 200 mg/kg showed reductions in the erythrocyte, haemoglobin and haematocrit values until the end of the study, and the numbers of reticulocytes and Heinz bodies were clearly increased 14 days after administration. These findings were interpreted by the authors as a slow development of anaemia which was probably made worse by increased degradation of the erythrocytes. The second animal in this dose group showed similar, but less marked, effects on the blood (Hoechst, 1988 f).

8.   Experience in humans

No information available.

9.   Threshold limit values

No information available.

References

Beilsteins Handbuch der organischen Chemie
4th Edition, Volume 12, p. 749
Springer, Berlin (1929)

Beilsteins Handbuch der organischen Chemie
4th Edition, 2nd supplement, Volume 12, E II 12, p. 406
Springer, Berlin Göttingen Heidelberg (1950)

Hoechst AG
Safety data sheet (1982)

Hoechst AG
Communication of 9. 8. 1984

Hoechst AG
2,4-Dinitromethylanilin – Prüfung auf Hautreizwirkung am Kaninchen
Report No. 88.0020 (1988 a)
Commissioned by BG Chemie

Hoechst AG
2,4-Dinitromethylanilin – Prüfung auf Augenreizwirkung am Kaninchen
Report No. 88.0045 (1988 b)
Commissioned by BG Chemie

Hoechst AG
2,4-Dinitromethylanilin – Prüfung der akuten oralen Toxizität an der Wistar Ratte
Report No. 88.0128 (1988 c)
Commissioned by BG Chemie

Hoechst AG
2,4-Dinitromethylanilin – Chromosome aberrations in vitro in V79 Chinese hamster cells
Report No. 88.0530 (1988 d)
Commissioned by BG Chemie

Hoechst AG
2,4-Dinitromethylanilin – Study of the mutagenic potential in strains of *Salmonella typhimurium* (Ames test) and *Escherichia coli*
Report No. 88.0713 (1988 e)
Commissioned by BG Chemie

Hoechst AG
2,4-Dinitromethylanilin – Wirkung auf das Blutbild an weiblichen Katzen
Report No. 88.0727 (1988 f)
Commissioned by BG Chemie

1,5-Naphthylene diamine

1.   Summary and assessment

1,5-Naphthylene diamine is of low acute toxicity (LD_{50} rat oral 2100 or 634 mg/kg, rat dermal >2000 mg/kg, LC_{50} rat inhalation $\geq$ 5270 mg/m^3/4 hours, LD_{50} rat subcutaneous 1563 mg/kg).

1,5-Naphthylene diamine does not irritate the skin and eyes.

This chemical shows sensitizing potential in the guinea-pig.

After repeated oral administration of 0.03 to 3% in the feed of rats and mice for 8 weeks, there are no characteristic symptoms of poisoning, but fatalities occur at concentrations of 0.3% or more.

1,5-Naphthylene diamine induces point-mutations in the Salmonella/microsome assay in strains TA 98, TA 100, TA 1537 and TA 1538, with and without metabolic activation (at concentrations of 200 to 300 µg/plate), but not in strain TA 1535, or in *Escherichia coli*. The chemical is not mutagenic in the HGPRT test on Chinese hamster V 79 cells, but in the presence of S9 mix it induces chromosomal aberrations at the highest test concentration of 150 µg/ml. In the UDS test for DNA-damaging effects on rat hepatocytes, no activity is evident at non-cytotoxic doses of 1.02–51.0 µg/ml. In general, these data show that 1,5-naphthylene diamine induces point-mutations and chromosomal damage in vitro. In vivo, however, there are no indications of DNA binding in rat liver.

Dietary administration to Fischer 344 rats for 103 weeks (0.1% and 0.05% 1,5-naphthylene diamine in the feed) causes a significant dose-related increase in the incidence of uterine polyps in the females. The incidence in the control group (approximately 8%) is relatively low compared with the spontaneous incidence (approximately 20%) reported in the literature for this rat strain. The relevance of the data reported must therefore be viewed with caution. An increased incidence of adenomas and carcinomas of the clitoral gland is found in the high dose group (0.1% in the feed), but this only reaches statistical significance ($p = 0.021$) if the adenomas and carcinomas are combined. The low-dose group showed no increase in tumours, although histological examination of the clitoral glands was only done where there were visible macroscopic changes, thus limiting the validity of this statement. No increase in the tumour incidence is seen in the male rats in this study, nor in male or female rats treated subcutaneously in a preliminary investigation.

In B6C3F1 mice, a dose-related increase in thyroid gland tumours is found in males and females, after 103 weeks of administering 0.2% and 0.1% 1,5-naphthylene diamine in the feed. In addition, there is a significant increase in the incidence of liver and lung tumours in female mice.

However, there were flaws in the experimental design of the chronic feeding study in rats and mice. There was no randomization in the allocation of animals to treated and untreated groups, and the observation period was 4 weeks longer in the controls than in the treated animals. The housing conditions were inadequate, as the temperature varied between 23 °C and 34 °C during the six air exchanges. Furthermore, several other feeding studies on mice and rats were in progress in the same room, some of them involving carcinogenic substances. The fact that, for example, only 78% of the male control mice could be histologically evaluated is an indication of inadequate care. Finally, it is significant that the histological examination of the clitoral glands was only carried out where there were visible macroscopic changes. Despite all these shortcomings, the results indicate possible carcinogenic activity in mice after high oral doses. The studies in rats do not permit a conclusion to be drawn on carcinogenic potential. A similar opinion is expressed in the IARC monograph on 1,5-naphthylene diamine ("The experiment in rats is inadequate for evaluation").

In strain A mice, 1,5-naphthylene diamine does not result in an increased incidence of lung tumours after intraperitoneal injection of a maximum dose of 25 mg/kg, three times a week for 8 weeks, with a post-observation period of 16 weeks. Nor is there any indication of carcinogenicity after life-time subcutaneous injections, giving a total dose of 7.55 g/kg.

2.   Name of substance

2.1   Usual name   1,5-Naphthylene diamine

2.2   IUPAC-name   1,5-Diaminonaphthalene

2.3   CAS-No.   2243-62-1

3.   Synonyms, common and trade names

1,5-Naphthyl diamine
1,5-Naphthalene diamine
1,5-Diaminonaphthalene
1,5-Naphthylendiamin

4.   Structural and molecular formulae

4.1 Structural formula

4.2 Molecular formula $C_{10}H_{10}N_2$

5.   Physical and chemical properties

5.1 Molecular mass, g/mol	158.2
5.2 Melting point, °C	189.5
5.3 Boiling point, °C	sublimates, some decomposes
5.4 Vapour pressure, hPa	2.3×10^{-8} hPa (at 20 °C) 2.2×10^{-6} hPa (at 50 °C) 1.67 hPa (at 190 °C)
5.5 Density, g/cm^3	0.996 (at 20 °C)
5.6 Solubility in water	0.04 g/l (at 20°C), soluble in hot water
5.7 Solubility in organic solvents	dissolves readily in ether, chloroform and hot alcohol
5.8 Solubility in fat	No information available
5.9 pH-value	ca. 6.8 at 0.04 g/l water
5.10 Conversion factor	1 ppm $\hat{=}$ 6.56 mg/m^3 1 mg/m^3 $\hat{=}$ 0.15 ppm (at 25 °C and 1013 hPa) (BAYER, 1989 a)

6.   Uses

Intermediate product for manufacturing azo dyes and isocyanates (Harnisch, 1979).

7.   Experimental results

7.1 Toxicokinetics and metabolism
No information available.

7.2 Acute and subacute toxicity
The acute oral toxicity of 1,5-naphthylene diamine as a preparation in polyethylene glycol 400 was tested on groups of ten male Wistar rats (strain TNO W74, average initial weight 170 g) with a single administration by stomach tube and an observation period of 14 days. The individual doses were not specified. The LD_{50} was calculated as 2100 (1860 to 2300) mg/kg (Probit slope factor 12.55). At toxic doses, the symptoms of poisoning included narcosis, shaggy fur, general malaise and weight loss. No effects were reported on macroscopic examination of some of the animals which died during the test or were killed at the end of the observation period (BAYER, 1981 a).

A similar test was carried out under the same conditions on groups of ten female Wistar rats (average initial weight 170 g). An LD_{50} of 634 (570 to 710) mg/kg was obtained (Probit slope factor 9.89). The symptoms of poisoning observed after the first week at toxic dose levels included narcosis, shaggy fur, general malaise and weight loss. Again, no effects were reported on macroscopic examination of some of the animals which died during the test or were killed at the end of the observation period (BAYER, 1981 b).

The acute subcutaneous toxicity of 1,5-naphthylene diamine, administered as an aqueous suspension, was tested on female Wistar-W.64 rats (120 to 140 g). The LD_{50} was 1563 mg/kg (1196 to 2185 mg/kg; nor further data; BAYER, 1974).

In order to test the acute dermal toxicity of 1,5-naphthylene diamine (purity 98.4%), a dose of 2000 mg/kg (combined in Cremophor EL) was applied once to the shaved skin of the back and flanks of five male and five female Wistar rats (average weight 253 and 197 g respectively). The application time was 24 hours, the observation period 14 days (Guideline 84/449/EEC; Official Journal of the European Communities No. L 251 of 19. 9. 1984, p. 103). No signs of systemic toxicity or of skin damage were observed, and all the animals survived. Subsequent examination of the animals that were killed after the observation period did not reveal any gross effects. Thus the dermal LD_{50} was >2000 mg/kg (BAYER, 1988 a).

The acute inhalation toxicity of 1,5-naphthylene diamine (purity 98.4%) was investigated in accordance with OECD Guideline no. 403 (1981) on five male and five female Wistar rats (average initial weight 170 to 200 g). The animals were exposed for 4 hours to the dust at concentrations of 2010 and 5270 mg/m^3. The mean mass-related aerodynamic particle diameter was 8.16 and 8.63 µm, respectively, with a geometric standard deviation of 2.39 and 2.26 µm, respectively. After exposure the animals were subsequently observed for 14 days. At a concentration of 2010 mg/m^3, there were no signs of poisoning and no deaths. At 5270 mg/m^3 the rats showed reduced motility, slower breathing and unkempt, ruffled fur. Two females died after 4 days, subsequent examination revealing fluid in the pleural cavity, reddened renal pelvis, dark and enlarged spleen, pallid liver with pattern of the lobes and reddened gastro-intestinal tract. Dissection of the rats killed after the observation period showed no recognisable lung damage, but in the females exposed to the higher concentration, the spleen was dark and enlarged. The LC_{50} of 1,5-naphthylene diamine was therefore >5270 mg/m^3 for male rats, and approx. 5270 mg/m^3 for female rats (BAYER, 1988 b).

7.3   Skin and mucous membrane effects

A test for primary skin irritation was carried out according to OECD test guideline no. 404 (1981) on three female albino rabbits (3.2 to 3.7 kg). 500 mg of 1,5-naphthylene diamine was mixed with water and applied semi-occlusively for 4 hours, and the rabbits were examined after 1, 24, 48 and 72 hours and after 7 days. In all the animals and at all observation times the average irritation value, according to Draize, was zero. 1,5-Naphthylene diamine therefore displayed no primary irritant effects on the skin (BAYER, 1986).

A test for eye irritation was carried out according to OECD test guideline no. 405 (1981) on three female albino rabbits (3.0 to 3.4 kg) with 100 µl (equivalent to approx. 100 mg) of 1,5-naphthylene diamine. After 24 hours the eyes were washed with physiological saline, and the findings evaluated after 1, 24, 48 and 72 hours and after 7 days. In all the animals and at all the observation times the average irritation value, according to Draize, was zero. Therefore 1,5-naphthylene diamine displayed no irritant effects on the eyes (BAYER, 1986).

7.4   Sensitization

1,5-Naphthylene diamine was tested for skin sensitization potential in the Magnusson and Kligman guinea-pig maximization test. A concentration of 2.5% in a formulation was used for intradermal induction and 50% for topical induction. The test sample was not primarily irritating at a concentration of 50%. The application site was therefore irritated with sodium lauryl sulphate prior to the topical induction. After the first challenge test with a concentration of 50%, skin reactions were seen in nine of the 20 animals (45%). The animals in the control group did not react. After this positive finding, a second challenge test was applied using lower concentrations, and a dose-dependent effect on the number of positively-reacting animals was observed. Ten animals (50%) reacted to the 25% test concentration, four animals (20%) to the 5% test concentration. The test sample therefore displayed a skin sensitising action in the maximization test on guinea-pigs, and must be regarded as a potential contact allergen for humans (BAYER, 1989 c).

7.5   Subchronic and chronic toxicity

In order to estimate the maximum tolerated dose of 1,5-naphthylene diamine in the feed for a long-term test, six groups of five male and five female Fischer-344 rats and B6C3F1 mice each received concentrations of 0, 0.03, 0.1, 0.3, 1.0 and 3.0% of the substance in the feed for 8 weeks. (The authors did not carry out a conversion to mg/kg body weight; according to the so-called Nelson Table, the respective values were approximately 20, 67, 200, 667 and 2000 mg/kg body weight/day for rats and 43, 143, 429, 1429 and 4286 mg/kg body weight/day for mice.) Mortality, clinical symptoms and weight gain were recorded (no further details). Deaths occurred amongst the rats given 0.3, 1.0 and 3.0% 1,5-naphthylene diamine in the feed (number and sex distribution not indicated), whilst at 0.1%, weight gain of the treated males and females was approximately 19% and 9% less than the controls, respectively. For rats, a concentration of 0.1% 1,5-naphthylene diamine in the feed was therefore chosen as the high dose level (maximum tolerated dose) for the long-term test. In male and female mice, deaths were also recorded at concentrations of 0.3% or more (number and sex distribution not indicated). Weight gain was depressed by 22% in males in the 0.3% dose group, but by only 3% in the females given the same dose. At 0.1%, the weight gain of the males was only 3% less than the controls. A concentration of 0.2% 1,5-naphthylene diamine in the feed was therefore chosen as the high dose level for mice in the long-term test. No data on any striking clinical symptoms is contained in the report (NCI, 1978).

7.6   Genotoxicity

7.6.1 In vitro
1,5-Naphthylene diamine showed dose-related mutagenic activity in strain TA 100 in the Salmonella/microsome test with and without activation by S9 mix from Aroclor-induced rat liver (showing a 2- to 3-fold increase in the number of revertants compared with the controls). At the tested doses of 3, 10, 33, 100, 333, 1000 and 3333 µg/plate, the lowest active dose was 333 µg/plate. In strains TA 1535, TA 1537, TA 1538 and TA 98, no mutagenic activity was demonstrable (no exact data). In the tested dose range, no cytotoxic effects were seen (Dunkel and Simmon, 1980).

The same authors carried out a spot test on the *Salmonella typhimurium* strains TA 98, TA 100, TA 1535, TA 1537and TA 1538, and the plate incorporation test on *Escherichia coli* WP2uvrA, at four independent institutes. The doses were between 0.3 and 3333.3 µg/plate, and the tests were carried out with and without metabolic activation (S9 mix from Aroclor 1254-induced livers of rats, mice and Syrian hamsters). 1,5-Naphthylene diamine (purity ≥96%) gave positive reactions (almost dose-dependent) on TA 98 and TA 1538 (with metabolic activation) and on TA 100 and TA 1537 (with and without metabolic activation). No point-mutagenic activity was evident in TA 1535 or in *Escherichia coli* (with or without metabolic activation). The results from the four institutes showed close agreement (Dunkel et al., 1985; Zeiger, 1987).

1,5-Naphthylene diamine (purity 98.4%) was tested in a further Salmonella/microsome test on strains TA 1535, TA 100, TA 1537 and TA 98, with and without metabolic activation (S9 mix from livers of rats pretreated with Aroclor 1254). In the preliminary test, concentrations ranging from 20 to 12,500 µg/plate were used. Concentrations at and above 2400 µg/plate showed a bacteriotoxic action. In the main test, doses of 300, 600, 1200, 2400, 4800 and 9600 µg/plate were used. In strains TA 100, TA 1537 and TA 98 there was a clear point-mutagenic effect with and without metabolic activation, at 300 µg/plate and above, whilst the results in TA 1535 were negative (BAYER, 1988 c).

A similar test was carried out with 1,5-naphthylene diamine (purity 99.2%). Here too there was clear mutagenic activity in strains

TA 100, TA 1537 and TA 98 from 200 µg/plate, with and without metabolic activation, the effect being greater with metabolic activation. Again, no positive effect was found in TA 1535 (BAYER, 1989).

In the HGPRT test (V 79 cells) at concentrations of 0.5, 1.0, 2.5 and 5.0 µg/ml without S9 mix and at 20, 50, 100 and 200 ng/ml and 150 µg/ml with S9 mix, no mutagenic activity was evident in two independent experiments. At the highest dose without S9 mix (5 µg/ml), 0.4 to 2.8% of the cells survived, and at the highest dose with S9 mix (150 µg/ml), 7.8 to 21.3% survived (LMP, 1986 a).

In an in vitro chromosome aberration test on V 79 cells of the Chinese hamster, the highest tested concentration (150 µg/ml) of 1,5-naphtylene diamine induced considerable chromosome damage and an increase in sister chromatid exchange, in the presence of S9 mix, after a treatment time of 28 hours (LMP, 1986 b).

In the UDS test, 1,5-naphthylene diamine (purity 98.4%) was tested for its DNA-damaging effect on primary rat hepatocytes. Concentrations of 102–1020 µg/ml were highly cytotoxic, so that only concentrations of 1.02–51.0 µg/ml (survival rate 97.7–62.9%) were tested. Within this concentration range, 1,5-naphthylene diamine had no effect on unscheduled DNA synthesis (Hazleton, 1988).

7.6.2 In vivo

In a DNA-binding study, two male Sprague-Dawley rats (approx. 220 g) received a single oral dose of 100 mg ^{3}H-labelled 1,5-naphthylene diamine (purity 98.8%)/kg ($\overset{\triangle}{=}$ 3.6 mCi/kg). The livers were extracted 24 hours later, the DNA and the chromatin protein were isolated and purified, and the specific radioactivity was measured. The recorded levels of 4.5 and 5.9 dpm/mg of DNA were slightly above normal. The covalent binding index averaged <0.2 (<0.18 and <0.23 respectively). For comparison, the covalent binding indices of 2-chloro-2-methylaniline and 4,4'-methylene-bis(2-chloro-aniline) were 9 and 28 respectively, under comparable conditions. According to the authors, these findings did not indicate any DNA binding activity of 1,5-naphthylene diamine (Institute of Toxicology, 1988).

7.7 Carcinogenicity

For the purpose of testing the carcinogenic activity of 1,5-naphthylene diamine, a long-term study was carried out on Fischer-344 rats and B6C3F1 mice. The animals were each 7 weeks old at the beginning of the study. 1,5-Naphthylene diamine was added to the feed at two concentrations; rats received 0.1 and 0.05% in the feed (the authors did not convert this to mg/kg, but according to the so-called Nelson table the values were approximately 33 and 67 mg/kg body weight/day, respectively), and mice received 0.2 and 0.1% in the feed (according to the so-called Nelson table, approximately 143 and 286 mg/kg body weight/day, respectively). For each concentration, 50 males and 50 females of each species were used, and the controls consisted of 50 male and 50 female mice and 25 male and 25 female rats. The substance was administered in the diet for 103 weeks, followed by an observation period of up to 4 weeks. The statistics were based on the Fisher-Exact test, the Cochram-Armitage test, etc. The doses administered did not affect the mortality of the rats or mice compared with their controls. The weight gain of the treated rats was equivalent to that of the controls, but in the treated mice a clear reduction in weight-gain was observed

Table1. Summary of the results of the NCI carcinogenicity study on rats

	Male rats			Female rats		
	Control	Low dose	High dose	Control	Low dose	High dose
Tumours of preputium or clitoris						
Number of animals tested	25	49	50	24	50	50
Carcinoma	0	0	1	1	3	8
Adenoma	0	0	1	0	0	5
Tumours of uterus and endometrium						
Number of animals tested	–	–	–	24	49	48
Polyps of the endometrium				2	14	20
Adenocarcinomas				1	2	4
Sarcomas of the endometrium				1	2	2

compared with the controls, the effect being more marked in males than in females. In the female rats of both dose groups, a statistically significant dose-dependent increase in stromatous polyps in the endometrium of the uterus was observed (see Table 1). These benign tumours occur relatively frequently in this strain of rat (Hasemann, 1983). The number of clitoral gland adenomas and carcinomas observed in female rats was only marginally significantly higher in the high-dose group compared with the controls (p=0.021). In both male and female rats, the incidence of tumours of the liver and thyroid gland was not significantly higher than in the controls. In male and female mice, a significant dose-related increase in thyroid

Table 2. Summary of the results of the NCI carcinogenicity study on mice

	Male mice			Female mice		
	Control	Low dose	High dose	Control	Low dose	High dose
Liver tumours						
Number of animals tested	39	45	43	46	49	46
Hepatocellular carcinomas	12	10	7	1	25	16
Hepatocellular adenomas	0	3	6	0	3	11
Thyroid gland tumours						
Number of animals tested	38	46	43	44	49	45
Follicle cell adenomas, papillomas and cystadenomas	0	8	16	2	17	14
C-cell adenomas	0	2	0	0	1	2
C-cell carcinomas	0	0	4	0	1	6
Lung tumours						
Number of animals tested	39	46	45	49	48	46
Alveolar/bronchiolar adenomas	2	6	2	0	9	2
Alveolar/bronchiolar carcinomas	2	3	0	0	1	3

gland tumours (papillomas, follicle cell adenomas, papillary cyst-adenomas) was observed in comparison with the controls (see Table 2). In addition, the female mice showed a significantly increased incidence of C-cell carcinomas, and of combined C-cell carcinomas and C-cell adenomas, of the thyroid gland. Moreover, the incidences of hepatocellular carcinomas and adenomas, and of adenomas or carcinomas of the lung in the alveolar and bronchiolar region, were significantly increased (NCI, 1978).

The relevance of the data reported must be viewed with caution due to flaws in the procedures during the performance of the studies.

Other authors subsequently used these results to calculate the median tumour-generating dose (TD_{50}) for the individual tumour types. The values obtained were 69.6 mg/kg body weight for uterine tumours in rats, 115 mg/kg body weight for liver tumours in female mice, 331 mg/kg body weight for lung tumours in female mice and 276 mg/kg body weight for thyroid gland tumours in male mice (Gold et al., 1986).

In an exploratory lifetime test involving subcutaneous administration of the maximum tolerated dose (up to a total dose of 7.55 g/kg) to 12 male and 12 female Wistar rats (control group of 25 males and 25 females) there was no indication of carcinogenic activity (BAYER, 1974).

1,5-Naphthylene diamine was also tested for its ability to induce lung tumours in strain A mice, a strain which is particularly susceptible to these tumours (spontaneous tumours appearing at the age of 3 to 4 months, the incidence after 24 months being almost 100%). Groups of ten male and female mice received intraperitoneal injections of 25, 12.5 or 6.25 mg/kg (in tricaprylin), three times per week for 8 weeks. The animals then remained untreated for a further 16 weeks. After a total of 24 weeks the tumour incidence was determined. No increase in the tumour rate (alveolar and bronchial adenomas) was observed relative to the controls. However, the authors pointed out that aromatic amines are generally only marginally active in this test (Maronpot et al., 1986).

In vitro

1,5-Naphtylene diamine was tested in the "survival test" for its cell-transforming properties. The criterion of cell transformation was the loss of contact inhibition of rat embryo cells ($2FR_450$) which were infected with Rauscher leukaemia virus. After 72 hours of incubation (37 °C) with 9.4 or 5.2 µg/5.2×10^4 cells, there was an increase in the survival rates of 213 and 106% respectively, relative to the controls, after a few days. This was evaluated as a positive finding (Traul et al., 1981).

7.8 Reproductive toxicity
No information available.

7.9 Effects on the immune system
No information available.

7.10 Neurotoxicity
No information available.

7.11 Other effects
No information available.

8.   Experience in humans

No information available.

9.   Threshold limit values

No information available.

References

BAYER AG, Institut of Toxicology
Orientierende Cancerogenese-Versuche mit subkutaner Gabe an Ratten
Unpublished report no. 5122 (1974)

BAYER AG, Institute of Toxicology
1,5-Naphthylendiamin subl. gem. (= Alphamin-1,5), Untersuchungen zur akuten oralen Toxizität an männlichen Wistar-Ratten
Unpublished report (1981 a)

BAYER AG, Institute of Toxicology
1,5-Naphthylendiamin subl. gem. (= Alphamin-1,5), Untersuchungen zur akuten oralen Toxizität an weiblichen Wistar-Ratten
Unpublished report (1981 b)

BAYER AG, Institute of Toxicology
1,5-Naphthylendiamin, Untersuchungen zum Reiz-/Ätzpotential an Haut und Augen (Kaninchen)
Unpublished report no. 14305 (1986)

BAYER AG, Institute of Toxicology
1,5-Naphthylendiamin, Untersuchungen zur akuten dermalen Toxizität an männlichen und weiblichen Wistar-Ratten
Unpublished report no. 16810 (1988 a)

BAYER AG, Institute of Toxicology
1,5-Naphthylendiamin, Untersuchungen zur akuten Inhalationstoxizität nach OECD-Richtlinie Nr. 403
Unpublished report no. 17320 (1988 b)

BAYER AG, Institute of Toxicology
1,5-Naphthylene diamine (not sublimated), Salmonella microsome test to evaluate for point-mutagenic effects
Unpublished report no. 17506 (1988 c)

BAYER AG
Grunddatensatz für Altstoffe, dated 6. 12. 1989 a

BAYER AG, Institute of Toxicology
1,5-Naphthylene diamine (sublimated and ground), Salmonella microsome test to evaluate for point-mutagenic effects
Unpublished report no. 17579 (1989 b)

BAYER AG, Institute of Toxicology
1,5-Naphthylendiamin – Untersuchungen auf hautsensibilisierende Wirkung bei Meerschweinchen
Unpublished report no. 18283 (1989 c)

Beilstein's Handbook of Organic Chemistry
Volume 13, 4th Edition, pp. 203–204
Springer, Berlin Heidelberg (1930)

Dunkel, V.C., Simmon, V.F.
Mutagenic activity of chemicals previously tested for carcinogenicity in the National Cancer Institute Bioassay Program
IARC Sci. Publ., 27, 283–302 (1980)

Dunkel, V.C., Zeiger, E., Brusick, D., McCoy, E., McGregor, D., Mortelmans, K., Rosenkranz, H.S., Simmon, V.F.
Reproducibility of microbial mutagenicity assays: II. Testing of carcinogens and non-carcinogens in *Salmonella typhimurium* and *Escherichia coli*
Environ. Mutagen., 7, Suppl. 5, 1–248 (1985)

Gold, L.S., Ward, J.M., Bernstein, L., Stern, B.
Association between carcinogenic potency and tumor pathology in rodent carcinogenesis bioassays
Fund. Appl. Toxicol., 6, 677–690 (1986)

Harnisch, H.
Napthalimid-Farbstoffe
In: Ullmanns Encyclopädie der technischen Chemie
4th edition, volume 17, p. 107–108
Verlag Chemie, Weinheim (1979)

Hasemann, J.K.
Patterns of tumor incidence in two year cancer bioassay feeding studies in Fisher 344 rats
Fund. Appl. Toxicol., 3, 1–9 (1983)

Hazleton Laboratories America, Inc.
Mutagenicity test on 1,5-naphthylene diamine (unsublimated) in the rat primary hepatocyte unscheduled DNA synthesis assay
Final Report to BAYER AG
Unpublished report no. R 4675 (1989)

IARC (International Agency for Research on Cancer)
Monographs on the evaluation of the carcinogenic risk of chemicals to humans
Vol. 27, 127–132 (1982)

Institute of Toxicology, Swiss Federal Institute of Technology and University of Zurich, CH-8603 Schwerzenbach, Switzerland
Investigation of the potential for covalent binding of 1,5-diamino-naphthalene to DNA of rat liver
Unpublished report commissioned by BG Chemie (1988)

Maronpot, R.R., Shimkin, M.B., Witschi, H.P., Smith, L.H., Cline, J.M.
Strain A mouse pulmonary tumor test results for chemicals previously tested in the National Cancer Institute carcinogenicity tests
J. Natl. Cancer Inst., 76, No. 6, 1101–1111 (1986)

LMP (Laboratorium für Mutagenitätsprüfungen)
Detection of gene mutations in somatic mammalian cells in culture: HGPRT-test with V 79 cells, Report LMP 141 A
Commissioned by BG Chemie, Heidelberg (1986 a)

LMP (Laboratorium für Mutagenitätsprüfungen)
Chromosome aberrations in cells of Chinese hamster cell line V 79,
Report LMP 141 B
Commissioned by BG Chemie, Heidelberg (1986 b)

NCI (National Cancer Institute)
Bioassay of 1,5-naphthylene diamine for possible carcinogenicity
Carcinogenesis Technical Report Series No. 143 (NCI-CG-TR-143)
(1978)

Traul, K.A., Takayama, K., Kachevsky, V., Hink, R.J., Wolff, J.S.
A rapid in vitro assay for carcinogenicity of chemical substances in
mammalian cells utilizing an attachment-independence endpoint, 2.
Assay validation
J. Appl. Toxicol., 1, No. 3, 190–195 (1981)

Zeiger, E.
Carcinogenicity of mutagens: predictive capability of the Salmonella
mutagenesis assay for rodent carcinogenicity
Cancer Res., 47, 1287–1296 (1987)

Compound chemical index vol. 1 and 2

Acetylene carbinol   *2*, 121
Acrylic acid   *2*, 41
Adipic acid dinitrile   *1*, 252
Adiponitrile   *1*, 252
Adipyl dinitrile   *1*, 252
AH   *1*, 182
2-Amino-1-methoxy-4-nitro-
   benzene   *1*, 155
1-Amino-2-methyl-4-nitroben-
   zene   *2*, 101
1-Amino-3-nitrobenzene   *2*, 88
1-Amino-4-chloro-2-nitroben-
   zene   *1*, 75
1-Amino-4-methoxy-2-methyl-
   benzene   *1*, 173
2-Amino-5-chloro-nitrobenzene
   1, 75
2-Amino-5-nitrotoluene   *2*, 101
2,2′-Aminodiethanol   *2*, 136
m-Aminonitrobenzene   *2*, 88
3-Aminonitrobenzene   *2*, 88
Ammonyx 200   *1*, 312
Ansibases Red RL   *2*, 101
asym-dimethyl ethylene
   2, 153
Azoamine Scarlet K   *1*, 155
Azoene Fast Red GL Base
   2, 101
Azogene Fast Red RL   *2*, 101
Azoic Diazo Component 13,
   Base   *1*, 155

1,4-Benzene dicarbonic acid
   dimethyl ester   *1*, 266
1,4-Benzene dicarboxylic acid
   dimethyl ester   *1*, 267
1,2-benzodicarbonitrile   *2*, 76

p-Benzoquinone monooxime
   2, 108
1,4-Benzoquinone oxime
   2, 108
N,N′-Bis(1-methylpropyl)-
   1,4-benzenediamine   *1*, 166
N,N′-Bis(1-methylpropyl)-
   1,4-diaminobenzene   *1*, 166
BLO   *1*, 134
Braunstein   *1*, 329
Brecolane NDG   *1*, 219
Butane dinitrile   *1*, 252
1,4-Butanolide   *1*, 134
But(2)ene-1,4-dicarboxylic acid
   dimethyl ester   *2*, 169
Butyl ethyl acetaldehyde
   2, 161
Butyl phosphate   *1*, 298
α-butylene   *2*, 153
γ-butylene   *2*, 153
i-butylene   *2*, 153
2-Butyne-1,4-diol   *1*, 207
Butynediol   *1*, 207
Butyric acid 4-hydroxy-,
   gamma-lactone   *1*, 134
Butyric acid lactone   *1*, 134
4-Butyrolactone   *1*, 134
Butyryl lactone   *1*, 134

CAEE   *1*, 319
CAS-No.
   75-02-5   *2*, 1
   78-83-1   *1*, 44
   78-79-5   *2*, 14
   79-07-2   *1*, 59
   79-10-7   *2*, 41
   89-63-4   *1*, 75

CAS-No.
91-15-6   *2*, 76
96-45-7   *1*, 83
96-48-0   *1*, 134
99-59-2   *1*, 155
99-09-2   *2*, 88
99-52-5   *2*, 101
101-96-2   *1*, 166
102-50-1   *1*, 173
104-76-7   *1*, 182
104-91-6   *2*, 108
107-19-7   *2*, 121
110-65-6   *1*, 207
111-42-2   *2*, 136
111-46-6   *1*, 219
111-69-3   *1*, 252
115-11-7   *2*, 153
120-61-6   *1*, 266
123-51-3   *1*, 284
123-05-7   *2*, 161
126-73-8   *1*, 298
138-24-9   *1*, 311
541-41-3   *1*, 319
624-48-6   *2*, 169
935-92-2   *2*, 178
1313-13-9   *1*, 328
2044-88-4   *2*, 185
2243-62-1   *2*, 192
Celluphos 4   *1*, 298
4-Chloro-2-nitroaniline   *1*, 75
Chloroacetamide   *1*, 59
α-Chloroacetamide   *1*, 60
2-Chloroacetamide   *1*, 59
Chloroacetic acid amide   *1*, 60
Chloroformic acid ethyl ester   *1*, 319
p-Chloro-o-nitroaniline   *1*, 75
C.I. 37030   *2*, 88
CNA   *1*, 75
m-Cresidine   *1*, 173

Daito Red Base RL   *2*, 101
DEA   *2*, 136
Deactivator E   *1*, 219
Deactivator H   *1*, 219
DEG   *1*, 219
Devol Red RL   *2*, 101
Diabase Red RL   *2*, 101
1,5-Diaminonaphthalene   *2*, 192
1,5-Diaminonaphthalene   *2*, 193
DICOL   *1*, 219
o-dicyanobenzene   *2*, 76
1,2-dicyanobenzol   *2*, 76
1,4-Dicyanobutane   *1*, 252
Diethanolamine   *2*, 136
N,N-Diethanolamine   *2*, 136
Diethylene glycol   *1*, 219
Diethylolamine   *2*, 136
Diglycol   *1*, 219
Dihydro-2(3H)-furanone   *1*, 133
4,5-Dihydro-2-mercap-toimidazole   *1*, 83
beta,beta'-Dihydroxydiethyl ether   *1*, 219
2,2'-Dihydroxy-diethylamine   *2*, 136
β,β'-Dihydroxy-diethylamine   *2*, 136
Dimethyl-1,4-benzene dicar-boxylate   *1*, 267
Dimethyl maleate   *2*, 169
Dimethyl terephthalate   *1*, 266
Dimethylmaleinat   *2*, 169
Dimethyl-p-phthalate   *1*, 267
2,4-Dinitro-1-methyl-amino-benzene   *2*, 185
2,4-Dinitromethylaniline   *2*, 185

2,4-Dinitro-N-methylaniline
   2, 185
But-2-yne-1,4-diol   *1*, 207
Diolamine   *2*, 136
1,4-Dioxy-butyne-2   *1*, 207
N,N′-Di-sec.-butyl-p-
   phenylenediamine   *1*, 166
Disflamol 1 TB   *1*, 298
Dissolvand APU   *1*, 219
DMM   *2*, 169
DMT   *1*, 267
DuPont Gasoline Antioxidant
   No. 22   *1*, 166

Ethanol, 2,2′-oxydi-   *1*, 219
Ethene carboxylic acid   *2*, 41
Z-Ethene dicarboxylic
   acid dimethyl ester   *2*, 169
Ethenyl methanol   *2*, 121
Ethylbutylacetaldehyde
   2, 162
2-Ethylcaproaldehyde   *2*, 161
α-Ethylcaproaldehyde   *2*, 162
Ethylchlorocarbonate   *1*, 319
Ethylchloroformiate   *1*, 319
Ethylchloromethanate   *1*, 319
Ethylene carboxylic acid   *2*, 42
Ethylene diglycol   *1*, 219
Ethylene thiourea   *1*, 83
Ethylenethiourea   *1*, 83
N,N′-Ethylenethiourea   *1*, 83
1,3-Ethylenethiourea   *1*, 83
Ethylhexaldehyde   *2*, 162
2-Ethylhexaldehyde   *2*, 162
2-Ethylhexan-1-ol   *1*, 182
2-Ethylhexanal   *2*, 161
2-Ethylhexanol-1   *1*, 182
2-Ethylhexanol   *1*, 182
2-Ethylhexyl alcohol   *1*, 182
Ethynyl carbinol   *2*, 121
ETU   *1*, 83

Fast Red 5NT   *2*, 101
Fast Red RL Base   *2*, 101
Fluoroethylene   *2*, 1

gamma-BL   *1*, 134
gamma-Butyrolactone   *1*, 133
GBL   *1*, 134
Glycol ether   *1*, 219
Glycol ethyl ether   *1*, 219
Golpanol   *1*, 207

Hemiterpene   *2*, 14
Hexanedioic acid dinitrile
   1, 252
Hiltonil Fast Red RL Base
   2, 102
1-Hydroxy-4-nitrosobenzene
   2, 108
4-Hydroxybutanoic acid lactone   *1*, 134
4-Hydroxybutanoic acid,
   gamma-lactone   *1*, 134
gamma-Hydroxybutyric acid
   cyclic ester   *1*, 134
gamma-Hydroxybutyric acid
   lactone   *1*, 134
4-Hydroxybutyric acid lactone   *1*, 134
4-Hydroxybutyric acid, gamma-
   lactone   *1*, 134
Bis-(2-hydroxyethyl)amine
   2, 136
Di-(2-hydroxyethyl)amine
   2, 136
Bis(2-hydroxyethyl)ether
   1, 219
1-Hydroxymethylpropane
   1, 44

Imidazolidinethione   *1*, 83
2-Imidazolidinethione   *1*, 83

Imidazoline-2(3H)-thione
  1, 83
Imidazoline-2-thiol *1*, 83
2,2′-Iminobisethanol *2*, 136
Isoamyl alcohol *1*, 284
Isobutanol *1*, 44
isobutene *2*, 153
Isobutyl alcohol *1*, 44
Isobutylcarbinol *1*, 284
isobutylene *2*, 153
Isoctanol *1*, 182
Isopentyl alcohol *1*, 284
Isoprene *2*, 14

Kako Red RL Base *2*, 102
Kayaku Red RL Base *2*, 102
Kerobit BPD *1*, 166
Korantin BH *1*, 207, 209

MAD *2*, 169
Maleic acid dimethyl ester
  2, 169
Manganese dioxide *1*, 328
Meisei Fast Red RL Base
  2, 102
2-Mercapto-2-imidazoline
  1, 83
Mercaptoimidazoline *1*, 83
Mercazin 1 NA 22 *1*, 83
4-Methoxy-2-methylaniline
  1, 173
4-Methoxy-2-methylbenzen
  amine *1*, 174
2-Methoxy-5-nitroaniline
  1, 155
2-Methoxy-5-nitrobenzen
  amine *1*, 155
Methyl-4-carbomethoxy-
  benzoate *1*, 267
2-Methyl-4-methoxyaniline
  1, 174

2-Methyl-4-nitroaniline *2*, 101
2-Methyl-4-nitrobenzenamine
  2, 101
2-Methyl-1,3-butadiene *2*, 14
N-Methyl-2,4-dinitroaniline
  2, 185
N-Methyl-2,4-dinitrobenzen-
  amine *2*, 185
β-Methyl bivinyl *2*, 14
Methyl maleate *2*, 169
Bis-oxy methylacetylene
  1, 207
Methylbutadiene-1,3 *2*, 14
3-Methylbutanol-1 *1*, 284
2-Methyl-p-anisidine *1*, 173
2-Methylpropan-1-ol *1*, 44
2-Methylpropane-1-ol *1*, 44
2-Methylpropanol-1 *1*, 44
2-Methylpropene *2*, 153
2-Methylpropyl alcohol *1*, 44
Microcide Mergal AF *1*, 60
2,2′-Iminodiethanol *2*, 136
Mitsui Red RL Base *2*, 102
Monofluoroethylene *2*, 1

1,5-Naphthalene diamine
  2, 193
1,5-Naphthyl diamine *2*, 193
1,5-Naphthylendiamin *2*, 193
1,5-Naphthylene diamine
  2, 192
Naphtoelan Red RL Base
  2, 102
NCI-C55878 *1*, 134
m-Nitranilin *2*, 88
5-Nitro-2-aminotoluene
  2, 101
m-Nitroaminobenzene *2*, 88
3-Nitroaniline *2*, 88
m-Nitroaniline *2*, 88
5-Nitroanisidine *1*, 155

3-Nitrobenzenamine   *2*, 88
5-Nitro-ortho-anisidine   *1*, 155
4-Nitro-o-toluidine   *2*, 101
p-Nitro-o-toluidine   *2*, 101
m-Nitrophenylamine   *2*, 88
p-Nitrosophenol   *2*, 108
4-Nitrosophenol   *2*, 108

Octanol, technical   *1*, 182
Octyl aldehyde   *2*, 162
3-Oxa-1,5-pentanediol   *1*, 219
3-Oxapentane-1,5-diol   *1*, 219
2,2′-Oxybisethanol   *1*, 220
2,2′-Oxydiethanol TL4N
   1, 220
o-PDN   *2*, 76

Pennac CRA   *1*, 83
Phenyltrimethyl-
   ammonium chloride   *1*, 311
Phosphoric acid tri-n-butyl-
   ester   *1*, 298
phthalic acid dinitrile   *2*, 76
o-phthalodinitrile (o-PDN)
   2, 76
phthalodinitrile   *2*, 76
Propargyl alcohol   *2*, 121
2-Propenoic acid   *2*, 42
Propyne-(1)-ol-(3)   *2*, 121
2-Propyne-1-ol   *2*, 121
Propyne-(2)-ol   *2*, 121
1-Propyne-3-ol   *2*, 121
2-Propynol-1   *2*, 121
p-Pseudocumoquinone
   2, 178
Pyrolusite   *1*, 329

p-Quinone monooxime
   2, 108
Quinone oxime   *2*, 108

Red Base Ciba X   *2*, 102
Red Base Irga X   *2*, 102
Red Base NRL   *2*, 102
Red RL Base   *2*, 102
Rhenogram ETU   *1*, 83
Rhodanin S 62   *1*, 83

Sipomer   *2*, 169
Soxinol 22   *1*, 83
Spectrolene Red RL   *2*, 102
Symulon Red RL Base   *2*, 102

TBP   *1*, 298
Tenamene 2   *1*, 166
Terephthalic acid dimethyl
   ester   *1*, 267
Tetramethylene cyanide
   1, 252
Tetramethylene dicyanide
   1, 252
Thiourea, N,N′-(1,2-ethan-
   diyl)   *1*, 83
Tributyl phosphate   *1*, 298
Tri-n-butyl phosphate   *1*, 298
2,3,5-Trimethyl-2,5-
   cyclohexadiene-1,4-dione
   2, 178
Trimethylanilinium chloride
   1, 312
N,N,N-Trimethylbenzen-
   ammonium chloride   *1*, 311
Trimethylbenzoquinone
   2, 178
Trimethylchinon   *2*, 178
2,3,5-Trimethylcyclohexa-2,5-
   diene-1,4-dione   *2*, 178
2,3,5-Trimethyl-p-benzo-
   quinone   *2*, 178
Trimethylphenyl ammonium
   chloride   *1*, 311
Trimethylquinone   *2*, 178

2,3,6-Trimethylquinone   *2*, 178
Tulabase Fast Red RL
   2, 102

VF   *2*, 1
Vinyl carboxylic acid   *2*, 42
Vinyl fluoride   *2*, 1

Vinyl fluoride   *2*, 2
Vulcacit NPV/C   *1*, 83

Warecure C   *1*, 83

Yamada Fast Red RL Base
   2, 102